INTRODUCTION TO RISK CALCULATION IN GENETIC COUNSELING

INTRODUCTION TO RISK CALCULATION IN GENETIC COUNSELING

Third Edition

Ian D. Young

Department of Clinical Genetics
Leicester Royal Infirmary
Leicester, United Kingdom

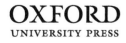
UNIVERSITY PRESS

2007

OXFORD
UNIVERSITY PRESS

Oxford University Press, Inc., publishes works that further
Oxford University's objective of excellence
in research, scholarship, and education.

Oxford   New York
Auckland   Cape Town   Dar es Salaam   Hong Kong   Karachi
Kuala Lumpur   Madrid   Melbourne   Mexico City   Nairobi
New Delhi   Shanghai   Taipei   Toronto

With offices in
Argentina   Austria   Brazil   Chile   Czech Republic   France   Greece
Guatemala   Hungary   Italy   Japan   Poland   Portugal   Singapore
South Korea   Switzerland   Thailand   Turkey   Ukraine   Vietnam

Published by Oxford University Press, Inc.
198 Madison Avenue, New York, New York 10016

www.oup.com

Oxford is a registered trademark of Oxford University Press

Library of Congress Cataloging-in-Publication Data
Young, Ian D.
Introduction to risk calculation in genetic counseling / Ian D. Young.—3rd ed.
p. ; cm.
Includes bibliographical references and index.
ISBN-13: 978-0-19-530527-2

1. Genetic counseling.   2. Health risk assessment.   3. Probabilities.   4. Genetic disorders—
Risk factors—Mathematical models.   I. Title.
[DNLM: 1. Genetic Counseling.   2. Risk Assessment. QZ 50
Y72i 2006]
RB155.7.Y68 2006
616'.042–dc22   2006001581

Printed in the United States of America
on acid-free paper

Preface

Although there has been remarkable progress in medical genetics over the past 10 years, with rapid advances in both molecular and computer technology, many situations still arise in which the providers of genetics services are called upon to undertake risk calculation. Indeed, the profusion of genetic tests has often served to fuel demand and expectations rather than ease this burden of responsibility. Factors such as heterogeneity, the use of linked markers, germline mosaicism, and the current limitations of mutation screening techniques have all served to complicate what was once perceived as a relatively straightforward process. In the present climate of accountability and litigation it is no longer acceptable, either in the clinic or in the laboratory, to conclude that a risk is simply high or low.

Numbers and probability theory are not to everyone's taste. Some genetic risks can be calculated easily. Others, to borrow a term from the popular pastime of Su Doku, can be fiendishly difficult. Those seeking guidance are not always helped by abstruse mathematical papers on the rigorous treatment of already difficult concepts. For most of us mere mortals, the maxim is to keep it short and simple. If it doesn't make sense to us, how can we hope to explain it to our colleagues or our patients? As with the two previous editions, this book has been written to come to the rescue of those who seek to master the basic principles without necessarily achieving grand master status.

Those who have access to the previous edition will note that there have been a number of significant changes. Case scenarios have been included in many chapters to further demonstrate how the theoretical principles can be applied in practice. Chapter 3 has been expanded to show how multiple consanguineous loops can be accommodated, and a new chapter has been included to address the difficult and very important issue of germline mosaicism. The chapters on cancer and multifactorial inheritance have been extensively revised, and a new appendix has been added to demonstrate approaches to the challenging calculations that can arise in prenatal diagnosis. Unfortunately, many publishers (Oxford University Press is a notable and worthy exception) now levy exorbitant fees to reproduce material from their books and journals, so that in some instances it has not been possible to include helpful illustrations and tables. It is hoped that readers will forgive this occasional omission, brought about by the importance of keeping the purchase price as low as possible.

Once again, I am indebted to the many colleagues who have reviewed relevant chapters and found embarrassing errors. Any that remain are entirely the responsibility of the author. Feedback from readers with comments and criticism, preferably constructive, is always welcome.

Contents

INTRODUCTION TO RISK CALCULATION
IN GENETIC COUNSELING

1

Genetic Counseling and the Laws of Probability

1.1 Genetic Counseling and the Concept of Risk

Genetic Counseling

Since the introduction of genetics clinics approximately 50 years ago, many attempts have been made to devise a universally acceptable definition of genetic counseling. As the subject has expanded, a consensus has gradually emerged that this should be viewed as a nondirective communication process that addresses an individual's needs and concerns relating to the development and/or transmission of a genetic disorder. This definition implies that the process of genetic counseling involves many important components, including the gathering of family information, the establishment of a diagnosis, the communication of information, and the provision of ongoing support. Equally important is the mathematical assessment of risk, and it is with this particular aspect of genetic counseling that this book is concerned.

It is true that in the past the determination of genetic risks often required little more than a knowledge of the basic principles of Mendelian inheritance. For many disorders, risk assessment simply involved the provision of a straightforward dominant or recessive recurrence risk, and today this still applies in some situations. However, an increasing awareness of the complexity and heterogeneity of genetic disease has focused attention on the importance of taking other factors, such as reduced penetrance and delayed age of onset, into account. In addition, the use of linked DNA markers and the increasing availability of specific mutation analysis often serve to complicate rather than simplify risk calculations that require careful consideration and a relatively high level of numerical competence if the provision of incorrect information is to be avoided.

3

Expressing a Risk in Mathematical Terms

There are several ways in which a risk can be expressed. Mathematically, probability is usually indicated as a proportion of 1, ranging from 0, indicating that an event cannot occur, up to 1, which implies that an event has to occur. However, many individuals are more comfortable with the concept of *odds*, as illustrated by the recent demonstration that a group of women being counseled for a family history of breast cancer actually expressed a preference for receiving information about risks in the form of "gambling odds" (Hopwood et al., 2003). Thus, a probability of 0.25 can be expressed as a risk of 1 in 4 ("1 chance in 4"), or 25%, that an event will occur, or conversely, as 3 chances out of 4 (75%) that an event will not occur. Note that a risk of 1 in 4 should not be expressed as 1:4, i.e., 1 *to* 4, which actually equals 1 *in* 5. When counseling those who are particularly comfortable with the concepts of gambling, a probability of 0.25 could also be expressed as odds of 3 to 1 against or 1 to 3 in favor of a particular outcome being observed.

Key Point 1

A probability or risk can be expressed

1. as a percentage, e.g., 50%
2. as a proportion of 1, e.g., 0.5
3. as a "chance," e.g., 1 chance in 2
4. as an odds ratio, e.g., 1 to 1 (evens)

Whilst discussing the quantitative nature of a risk, it is both helpful and important to point out that chance does not have a memory. The fact that a couple's first child has an autosomal recessive disorder does not imply that their next three children will be unaffected. The key point is that the risk of 1 in 4 applies to *each* future child. It can be extremely embarrassing to learn that a second affected child has been born to parents who have clearly misinterpreted information given at a previous counseling session.

Qualifying a Genetic Risk

The provision of a genetic risk does not simply involve the conveyance of a risk figure in stark isolation. Genetic risks should be qualified in a number of ways. For example, risks should be placed in context, perhaps by pointing out that 1 in 40 of all babies has a congenital malformation when dealing with a pediatric problem, or by reminding adults at risk of malignancy that there is an extremely high background population risk of approximately 1 in 3 for developing cancer. It is also important that the genetic counselor should not be seen exclusively as a prophet of doom. Thus, it is well worth emphasizing that a risk of 1 in 20 for an adverse outcome such as a neural tube defect means that there are 19 chances out of 20 that a future baby will not be affected.

Having ensured that a risk has been correctly quantified, understood, and placed in context, it is essential that an indication should be given of what the risk is actually for. Does the quoted figure relate to the risk of inheriting the relevant gene or does it give an indication of the probability that a serious complication will occur? The interpretation of severity and risk is subjective and unpredictable. For example, some parents who have undergone extensive surgery in childhood for repair of an abnormality such as cleft lip and palate can be profoundly concerned about a relatively low polygenic/multifactorial risk for offspring. In contrast, other prospective parents with disorders such as achondroplasia or autosomal dominant deafness are often not at all perturbed by much higher risks for offspring. In some genetics text books it is stated that, as an arbitrary guide, risks of 1 in 10 or greater can be viewed as "high," 1 in 20 or less as "low," and intermediate values as "moderate." As a generalization, these values have some merit, but for many individuals the perception and interpretation of risk are based more on emotion and personal experience than on cold objectivity and logic. Studies of the long-term impact of genetic counseling have shown that it is the burden of a disorder rather than its precise risk that is of major concern to counselees.

This brings us to a final point that is often raised in the context of risk calculation. A case can reasonably be made that many counselees are primarily concerned with whether a risk is high or low, and that it is therefore both unnecessary and unhelpful to define a risk to the nearest decimal point. While this may well be true in some situations, it does not detract from the importance of giving correct and precise information, an obligation neatly summarized by Lalouel et al. as long ago as 1977, when they maintained that "the question of whether consultees demand as much specificity should be subordinate to the question of whether counselors are justified in providing less." Almost 30 years later, in an editorial in the *American Journal of Medical Genetics* (Hodge and Flodman, 2004), the point was elegantly made that it can be extremely dangerous to "trust intuition," as illustrated by estimated carrier risks ranging from less than 1% to 50% for a specific female in a cited X-linked pedigree—the correct value was 10.7% (Hodge and Flodman, 2005). There is some evidence that it is more effective to present risks in the form of numbers rather than words (Marteau et al., 2000), and it is obvious that if a numerical risk is being given, then it should be correct.

1.2 The Laws of Probability

Two relatively simple principles are often used when calculating risks in genetic counseling. These are known as the *laws of addition and multiplication*.

Law of Addition

If two (or more) events are mutually exclusive, and the probability of event one occurring is $P1$ and that of event two occurring is $P2$, then the probability of *either* the first event *or* the second event occurring equals $P1 + P2$. An obvious example of the application of this law is the probability that a baby will be male or female. If the probability of having a boy equals 0.5 and the probability of having a girl also equals 0.5, then the probability that any particular baby will be *either* male *or* female equals 1.

Law of Multiplication

This law is applied when the outcome of two (or more) events is independent. If the probability of one event occurring is $P1$ and that of another event is $P2$, then the probability of *both* the first *and* the second event occurring equals $P1 \times P2$. For example, if parents are considering having two children, then excluding the unlikely event of identical twins, the probability that both children will be boys equals the product of the probabilities that *both* the first child *and* the second child will be male, i.e., $1/2 \times 1/2 = 1/4$.

Key Point 2

Probabilities are added when they relate to mutually exclusive alternative outcomes. Probabilities are multiplied when they relate to independent events or outcomes.

Examples Based on Twin Pregnancies

The demonstration of twins in a pregnancy can generate some difficult counseling problems (Hunter and Cox, 1979). The following two examples show how these simple laws of addition and multiplication can be used to calculate the probability that one or both babies will be affected with a genetic disorder. The underlying principle is to determine the probabilities if the twins are either monozygotic (MZ) or dizygotic (DZ) and then calculate the total risks by adding the probabilities for each weighted on the basis of their relative frequencies. In these examples, it is assumed that the ratio of MZ to DZ twinning is 1 to 2, i.e., that one-third of twin pairs are MZ and two-thirds are DZ.

Example 1

Healthy parents have had a child with a severe autosomal recessive disorder. Aware of the recurrence risk of 1 in 4, they embark upon another pregnancy. During the early stages of this pregnancy, ultrasonography reveals the presence of twins. The parents now wish to know the probability that at least one twin will be affected by the autosomal recessive disorder.

To answer this question, the risks are first calculated for the two mutually exclusive possibilities that the twins are either (1) monozygotic ($P = 1/3$) or (2) dizygotic ($P = 2/3$).

1. Monozygotic. In this situation, the probability that both twins will be affected equals 1/4, that only one will be affected equals 0, and that both will be unaffected equals 3/4.

2. Dizygotic. If the twins are dizygotic, then the genotype of one twin does not influence the genotype of the other twin, i.e., these events are independent. Therefore, the probability that both twins will be affected equals 1/16 (i.e., $1/4 \times 1/4$), the probability that only one will be affected equals 3/8 [i.e., $(1/4 \times 3/4) + (3/4 \times 1/4)$], and the probability that both will be unaffected equals 9/16 (i.e., $3/4 \times 3/4$).

Using this combination of mutually exclusive and independent events, the parents' question can now be answered. The overall probability that

1. both twins will be affected equals MZ ($1/3 \times 1/4$) plus DZ ($2/3 \times 1/16$), giving a total probability of 1/8.
2. only one twin will be affected equals MZ ($1/3 \times 0$) plus DZ ($2/3 \times 3/8$), giving a total probability of 1/4.
3. both twins will be unaffected equals MZ ($1/3 \times 3/4$) plus DZ ($2/3 \times 9/16$), giving a total probability of 5/8.

Based on this information, the parents can be reliably informed that there is a probability of $1/8 + 1/4 = 3/8$ that at least one of their unborn babies will be affected.

Example 2

A healthy 40-year-old woman with no relevant family history is found to be carrying twins and wishes to know the probability that one or both of her babies will have Down syndrome. In calculating the answer, it is assumed that the ratio of MZ to DZ twinning remains constant at 1:2 at all ages and that the risk of Down syndrome in a singleton pregnancy conceived by a 40-year-old woman equals 1 in 100.

Once again, the first step is to determine the risks for each of the two mutually exclusive possibilities, i.e., that the twins are either monozygotic or dizygotic.

1. Monozygotic. The probability that both twins will be affected equals 1/100, that only one will be affected equals 0 (this ignores the unlikely possibility of postzygotic nondisjunction), and that both will be unaffected equals 99/100.
2. Dizygotic. The karyotypes of the twins are independent of each other. Therefore, the probability that both will be affected equals 1/10 000 (i.e., $1/100 \times 1/100$), the probability that only one twin will be affected equals 198/10 000 (i.e., $2 \times 1/100 \times 99/100$), and the probability that both will be unaffected equals 9801/10,000 (i.e., $99/100 \times 99/100$).

The concluding step is to weight the probabilities obtained, assuming either MZ or DZ according to their relative frequencies, i.e., 1:2. The overall probability that

1. both twins will be affected equals MZ ($1/3 \times 1/100$) plus DZ ($2/3 \times 1/10,000$)), which equals 17/5000 (approximately 1 in 294 or 0.34%).
2. only one twin will be affected equals MZ ($1/3 \times 0$) plus DZ ($2/3 \times 198/10,000$), which equals 66/5000 (approximately 1 in 76 or 1.32%).
3. both twins will be unaffected equals MZ ($1/3 \times 99/100$) plus DZ ($2/3 \times 9801/10,000$), which equals 4917/5000 or 98.34%.

Based on this information, the prospective mother can be informed that the probability that at least one of the twins will have Down syndrome equals 1.66% or 1 in 60.

1.3 The Binomial Distribution

Use of the binomial distribution enables easy calculation of the probability of obtaining a particular number or distribution of events of one kind (e.g., boys or girls) in a sample, given knowledge of the probability of each event occurring independently. The binomial distribution can be presented in the form of an equation.

$$P = \frac{n!}{(n-r)!r!}p^{n-r}q^r$$

where

$P =$ the probability of observing the particular split of r of one event and $n - r$ of the other
$n =$ the total sample size
$r =$ the number of events of one type observed
$p =$ the probability of this event not occurring
$q =$ the probability of this event occurring
$! =$ factorial, e.g., $4! = 4 \times 3 \times 2 \times 1$, and by convention $0! = 1$

Example 3

Prospective parents who are planning to decorate their spare bedrooms wish to know the probability that their prenatally diagnosed quadruplets will consist of both boys and girls. To simplify the calculation, it is assumed that the babies were conceived with the help of an ovulation-inducing drug such as clomiphene, so that the probability that they are MZ can effectively be ignored.

In this example, the sibship size (n) equals 4, and the probability of a male baby (p) equals the probability of a female baby (q) equals 1/2. Using the binomial distribution, the probability of having zero, one, two, three, or four male babies can be calculated as follows:

1. no male babies

$$P = \left(\frac{1}{2}\right)^4 = \frac{1}{16}$$

2. one male baby ($r = 1$)

$$P = \frac{4!}{3! \ 1}\left(\frac{1}{2}\right)^3\frac{1}{2} = \frac{1}{4}$$

3. two male babies ($r = 2$)

$$P = \frac{4!}{2! \ 2!}\left(\frac{1}{2}\right)^2\left(\frac{1}{2}\right)^2 = \frac{3}{8}$$

4. three male babies ($r = 3$)

$$P = \frac{4!}{1! \ 3!} \left(\frac{1}{2}\right)^1 \left(\frac{1}{2}\right)^3 = \frac{1}{4}$$

5. four male babies

$$P = \left(\frac{1}{2}\right)^4 = \frac{1}{16}$$

Thus, these parents can be informed that there is a probability of

$$\frac{\frac{1}{4} + \frac{3}{8} + \frac{1}{4}}{\frac{1}{16} + \frac{1}{4} + \frac{3}{8} + \frac{1}{4} + \frac{1}{16}} = \frac{7}{8}$$

that their quadruplets will consist of different-sex infants.

Example 4

In this example the same prospective parents are expecting nonidentical quadruplets, having already had a child with an autosomal recessive disorder. They wish to know the probability that at least two of their four babies will be affected.

The calculation proceeds as in Example 3, but now $p = 3/4$ and $q = 1/4$, i.e.:

1. no affected babies

$$P = \left(\frac{3}{4}\right)^4 = \frac{81}{256}$$

2. one affected baby ($r = 1$)

$$P = \frac{4!}{3! \ 1} \left(\frac{3}{4}\right)^3 \frac{1}{4} = \frac{108}{256}$$

3. two affected babies ($r = 2$)

$$P = \frac{4!}{2! \ 2!} \left(\frac{3}{4}\right)^2 \left(\frac{1}{4}\right)^2 = \frac{54}{256}$$

4. three affected babies ($r = 3$)

$$P = \frac{4!}{1} \frac{3}{3! 4} \left(\frac{1}{4}\right)^3 = \frac{12}{256}$$

5. four affected babies

$$P = \left(\frac{1}{4}\right)^4 = \frac{1}{256}$$

Thus, these parents can be informed that the probability that at least two of their four babies will be affected equals

$$\frac{54 + 12 + 1}{81 + 108 + 54 + 12 + 1} = \frac{67}{256}$$

Example 5

The binomial distribution can be used in many other situations, such as that outlined in Chapter 3 (p. 53), in which parents have had children affected with different auto-somal recessive disorders. In this example, consider parents who have already had three children, each with a different autosomal recessive disorder. They wish to know the probabilities that their next child will inherit all, some, or none of these conditions. To simplify matters, it is assumed that the loci of the disorders are not linked. The various probabilities can be calculated using the binomial distribution, where

n = the total number of disorders
r = the number of disorders inherited by the fourth child
p = the probability of not inheriting each disease = 3/4
q = the probability of inheriting each disease = 1/4

Thus, the probabilities for the next child will be

1. child inherits none of the conditions

$$P = \left(\frac{3}{4}\right)^3 = \frac{27}{64}$$

2. child inherits one condition ($r = 1$)

$$P = \frac{3!}{2! \; 1} \left(\frac{3}{4}\right)^2 \frac{1}{4} = \frac{27}{64}$$

3. child inherits two conditions ($r = 2$)

$$P = \frac{3!}{1 \; 2!} \frac{3}{4} \left(\frac{1}{4}\right)^2 = \frac{9}{64}$$

4. child inherits all three conditions ($r = 3$)

$$P = \left(\frac{1}{4}\right)^3 = \frac{1}{64}$$

Key Point 3

The binomial distribution is obtained by expanding $(p + q)^n$ and can be used to determine the probability that a particular distribution of events (e.g., boys or girls, heads or tails) will occur.

Pascal's Triangle

The binomial distribution is derived by expanding $(p + q)^n$. This can be presented diagrammatically in the form of a triangle, which derives its name from the famous French mathematician and polymath Blaise Pascal.

Sample Size $(=n)$	Expansion of $(p+q)^n$	Number of Possible Combinations
1	$p \quad q$	2
2	$p^2 \quad 2pq \quad q^2$	3
3	$p^3 \quad 3p^2q \quad 3pq^2 \quad q^3$	4
4	$p^4 \quad 4p^3q \quad 6p^2q^2 \quad 4pq^3 \quad q^4$	5
5	$p^5 \quad 5p^4q \quad 10p^3q^2 \quad 10p^2q^3 \quad 5pq^4 \quad q^5$	6
n	$p^n \quad np^{n-1}q \quad \cdots \quad npq^{n-1} \quad q^n$	$n+1$

The number preceding each term in the triangle is known as the *coefficient of the expansion* and can be obtained easily by adding together the two coefficients lying on either side of it in the row above. This coefficient is equal to $\frac{n!}{(n-r)!r!}$ in the equation, which defines the binomial distribution. Thus, those who dislike algebra intensely can use Pascal's triangle rather than the full binomial distribution. For example, if parents who both carry the same autosomal recessive gene have five children, they might wish to know the probability that three will be affected. Using the binomial distribution, the answer will be

$$\frac{5!}{2! \ 3!} \left(\frac{3}{4}\right)^2 \left(\frac{1}{4}\right)^3 = \frac{90}{1024}$$

The same answer can be obtained by consulting Pascal's triangle and reading across the line $n = 5$. The coefficient for $p^2 q^3$ (i.e., 2 unaffected and 3 affected) is 10. Thus, the desired probability will be $10 \times \left(\frac{3}{4}\right)^2 \times \left(\frac{1}{4}\right)^3 = \frac{90}{1024}$.

1.4 Bayes' Theorem

This theorem provides an extremely useful means of quantifying genetic risks (Murphy and Mutalik, 1969). It is derived from an essay on the *doctrine of chances* written by an eighteenth-century English clergyman, Thomas Bayes, first published posthumously by one of his friends in 1763 and republished in 1958 (Bayes, 1958). Essentially, it offers a method for considering all possibilities or events and then modifying the probabilities for each of these by incorporating information that sheds light on which is the most likely. The initial probability for each event, such as being a carrier or not being a carrier, is known as its *prior* probability and is based on "anterior" information such as the ancestral family history. The observations that modify the prior probabilities allow *conditional* probabilities to be derived using "posterior" information such as the results of carrier tests.

The resulting probability for each possibility or event is known as its *joint* probability and is calculated by multiplying the prior probability by the conditional probability for each observation (the observations should be independent in that they should not influence each other). The overall final probability for each event is known as its *posterior* or *relative* probability and is obtained by dividing its joint probability by the sum of all of the joint probabilities. This has the effect of ensuring that the sum of all of the posterior probabilities always equals 1. Alternatively, posterior probabilities can be expressed in the form of odds for or against a particular event occurring or not occurring.

On first reading this can be very confusing, and the reader will not necessarily be helped by the following formal statement of Bayes' theorem:

1. If the prior probability of an event C occurring is denoted as $P(C)$ and
2. the prior probability of event C not occurring is denoted as $P(NC)$ and
3. the conditional probability of observation O occurring if C occurs equals $P(O|C)$ and
4. the conditional probability of observation O occurring if C does not occur equals $P(O|NC)$, then the overall probability of event C given that O is observed equals

$$\frac{P(C) \text{ multiplied by } P(O|C)}{[P(C) \text{ multiplied by } P(O|C)] + [P(NC) \text{ multiplied by } P(O|NC)]}$$

This may be a little clearer if a Bayesian table (Table 1.1) is constructed. The posterior probability of event C occurring equals

$$\frac{P(C) \times P(O|C)}{[P(C) \times P(O|C)] + [P(NC) \times P(O|NC)]}$$

The posterior probability of event C not occurring equals

$$\frac{P(NC) \times P(O|NC)}{[P(C) \times P(O|C)] + [P(NC) \times P(O|NC)]}$$

This is not nearly as complicated or difficult as it seems. If you are not convinced, then consider the following example.

Example 6

A woman, II2 in Figure 1.1, wishes to know the probability that she is a carrier of Duchenne muscular dystrophy. Her concern is based upon her family history, which reveals an affected brother and an affected maternal uncle. This is anterior information that enables the prior probability that she is a carrier $P(C)$ to be de-

Table 1.1.

Probability	Event C Occurs	Event C Does Not Occur
Prior	$P(C)$	$P(NC)$
Conditional O occurs	$P(O|C)$	$P(O|NC)$
Joint	$P(C) \times P(O|C)$	$P(NC) \times P(O|NC)$

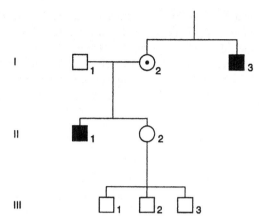

Figure 1.1. When calculating the probability that II2 is a carrier of Duchenne muscular dystrophy Bayes' theorem provides a method for taking into account the fact that she already has three unaffected sons.

termined. As her mother (I2) must be a carrier, there is a prior probability of 1/2 that II2 is a carrier and an equal prior probability of 1/2 that she is not a carrier.

Posterior information is provided by the fact that the consultand already has three unaffected sons. If the consultand is a carrier, then each of her sons will have a risk of 1 in 2 of being affected. Thus, $P(O|C)$ equals $1/2 \times 1/2 \times 1/2$ since the consultand has three unaffected sons, and $P(O|NC)$ equals $1 \times 1 \times 1$, since if the consultand is not a carrier, there is a probability of 1 $(1 - \mu$, to be exact, but μ—the mutation rate—can be ignored since it is less than 1/1000) that a son will be unaffected.

This information is used to construct a Bayesian table (Table 1.2). The posterior probability that the consultand is a carrier equals $1/16/(1/16 + 1/2)$, which equals 1/9. Alternatively, the posterior probability can be stated in the form of odds by indicating that there are 8 chances to 1 that the consultand is not a carrier.

Effectively, in this example Bayes' theorem has been used to quantify the intuitive recognition that the birth of three unaffected sons makes it rather unlikely

Table 1.2.

Probability	Consultand Is a Carrier		Consultand Is Not a Carrier
Prior	$\dfrac{1}{2}$		$\dfrac{1}{2}$
Conditional 3 unaffected sons	$\dfrac{1}{8}$		1
Joint	$\dfrac{1}{16}$		$\dfrac{1}{2}$
Odds	1	to	8

Posterior probability that consultand is a carrier $= \dfrac{\frac{1}{16}}{\frac{1}{16} \times \frac{1}{2}} = \dfrac{1}{9}$

Posterior probability that consultand is not a carrier $= \dfrac{\frac{1}{2}}{\frac{1}{16} \times \frac{1}{2}} = \dfrac{8}{9}$

that the consultand is a carrier. The greater the number of unaffected sons, then, the more likely it becomes that the consultand is not a carrier. Obviously, the birth of one affected son would totally negate the conditional probability contributed by unaffected sons by introducing conditional probabilities of 1/2 (carrier) versus μ (new mutation) in the noncarrier column. In other words, the birth of an affected son would make it overwhelmingly likely that the consultand is a carrier.

Key Point 4

Bayes' theorem provides a method for taking into account all relevant information when calculating the probability of an event such as carrier status. Key points to remember are:

1. A table should be drawn up that includes all relevant possibilities.
2. The prior probability for each possibility is derived from ancestral anterior information.
3. The conditional probabilities are obtained from posterior information that sheds light on which initial possibility is more or less likely. Conditional probabilities can be calculated by asking "What is the probability that this observation would be made given that the initial possibility or event occurs or applies?"
4. The joint probability for each possibility is calculated and then compared with the other joint probabilities to give a posterior or relative probability for each possibility or event.
5. All relevant information should be used once and only once.

The concepts introduced in this chapter, and in Bayes' theorem in particular, are not easy to grasp. However, with a little practice, even the most reluctant mathematician can become reasonably proficient at simple probability calculations. More testing examples are provided in the next four chapters. Readers who are still struggling with the underlying principles are invited to consult the review by Ogino and Wilson (2004), which provides a very clear explanation of how to apply Bayesian analysis.

1.5 Case Scenario

A woman, II2 in Figure 1.2, is referred from the antenatal clinic for genetic risk assessment. She is 20 weeks pregnant and is known to have two maternal uncles and a brother with severe learning disability. Investigations undertaken in the past, including Fragile X mutation analysis, have failed to identify a specific cause, prompting a clinical diagnosis of nonspecific X-linked mental retardation. Ultrasonography has revealed that this woman is carrying male twins (III2 and III3) of unknown zygosity. The woman specifically wishes to know the probability that one or both of her unborn sons will be affected.

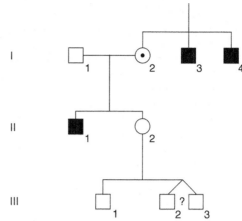

Figure 1.2. II2 is carrying male twins of unknown zygosity. What is the probability that none, one, or both will be affected?

To answer her question, we have to carry out three relatively easy calculations using two Bayesian tables and a simple application of the basic laws of probability.

1. The first Bayesian calculation (Table 1.3) indicates the probability that this woman is a carrier of the X-linked mental retardation that affects her uncles and brother. This yields a figure of 1 in 3, which is less than the ancestral prior pedigree risk of 1 in 2 because the woman already has an unaffected son (III1).

2. The second Bayesian calculation (Table 1.4) determines the probability that the male twins are either MZ or DZ, given that the ratio of MZ to DZ twins is 1:2. As shown in Table 1.4, half of all same-sex twins will be MZ and half will be DZ.

Table 1.3.*

Probability	II2 Is a Carrier	II2 Is Not a Carrier
Prior	$\frac{1}{2}$	$\frac{1}{2}$
Conditional		
1 unaffected son	$\frac{1}{2}$	1
Joint	$\frac{1}{4}$	$\frac{1}{2}$
Odds	1 to	2

Posterior probability that II2 is a carrier $= \frac{1}{4} \Big/ \left(\frac{1}{4} + \frac{1}{2}\right) = \frac{1}{3}$

Posterior probability that II2 is not a carrier $= \frac{1}{2} \Big/ \left(\frac{1}{4} + \frac{1}{2}\right) = \frac{2}{3}$

*See Figure 1.2.

Table 1.4.

Probability	Twins Are MZ		Twins Are DZ
Prior	$\frac{1}{3}$		$\frac{2}{3}$
Conditional (same sex)	1		$\frac{1}{2}$
Joint	$\frac{1}{3}$		$\frac{1}{3}$
Odds	1	to	1

Posterior probability that the twins are MZ $= \dfrac{1}{3} \bigg/ \left(\dfrac{1}{3}+\dfrac{1}{3}\right) = \dfrac{1}{2}$

Posterior probability that the twins are DZ $= \dfrac{1}{3} \bigg/ \left(\dfrac{1}{3}+\dfrac{1}{3}\right) = \dfrac{1}{2}$

Note that conditional probabilities of $\frac{1}{2}$ and $\frac{1}{4}$ for both twins being boys could also be used. These would yield joint probabilities of $\frac{1}{6}$ and $\frac{1}{6}$, giving the same posterior probabilites of 1/2 and 1/2 for being MZ or DZ.

3. We now calculate the probability that none, one, or both of the twins will be affected given that there is 1 chance in 3 that their mother is a carrier and that there is an equal chance that the twins are MZ or DZ.

a. The probability that neither twin will be affected equals:

2/3 (the probability that II2 is not a carrier)

$\times 1, + 1/3$ (the probability that II2 is a carrier)

$\times [\text{MZ } (1/2 \times 1/2) + \text{DZ } (1/2 \times 1/4)],$

which equals $2/3 + 1/3(1/4 + 1/8), = 19/24.$

b. The probability that one twin will be affected equals:

$2/3 \times 0, + 1/3 \times [\text{MZ } (1/2 \times 0) + \text{DZ } (1/2 \times 1/2)],$

which equals 1/12.

c. The probability that both twins will be affected equals:

$2/3 \times 0, + 1/3 \times [\text{MZ } (1/2 \times 1/2) + \text{DZ}(1/2 \times 1/4),$

which equals 1/8.

Therefore, the probability that at least one twin will be affected equals $1/12 + 1/8 = 5/24.$

Further Reading

Emery, A.E.H. (1986). *Methodology in medical genetics* (2nd ed.). Churchill Livingstone, Edinburgh.

Harper, P.S. (2004). *Practical genetic counselling* (6th ed.). Arnold, London.

Hodge, S.E. (1998). A simple unified approach to Bayesian risk calculations. *Journal of Genetic Counseling*, **7,** 235–261.

Mould, R.F. (1998). *Introductory medical statistics* (3rd ed.). Institute of Physics, Bristol and Philadelphia.

Murphy, E.A. and Chase, G.A. (1975). *Principles of genetic counseling*. Year Book Medical Publishers, Chicago.

Ogino, S. and Wilson, R.B. (2004). Bayesian analysis and risk assessment in genetic counseling and testing. *Journal of Molecular Diagnostics*, **6,** 1–9.

2

Autosomal Dominant Inheritance

Disorders that show autosomal dominant inheritance are caused by mutations in genes located on one of the autosomes and are manifest in heterozygotes. The calculation of risks for these disorders is generally straightforward, particularly if there is a clear family history and the disorder in question is characterized by complete penetrance, consistent expression, and a reliable means of diagnosis. The probability that each child of an affected individual will inherit the condition is 1 in 2 (50%), whereas the child of an unaffected family member will be at negligible risk or, more precisely, twice the mutation rate (i.e., 2μ, where $\mu =$ the mutation rate per gamete per generation).

However, in many situations, risk calculation for autosomal dominant inheritance can prove to be much more complex than might initially be anticipated. Several factors, such as reduced penetrance, age-dependent penetrance, homozygosity, and anticipation can significantly influence the final risk. These various factors are considered in the following pages.

2.1 Reduced Penetrance

A disorder is said to show reduced *penetrance* when it has clearly been demonstrated that individuals who must carry the abnormal gene, and are therefore referred to as *obligatory heterozygotes*, show absolutely no phenotypic manifestations of its effects. Thus, if someone who is totally unaffected has a parent and a child with a particular autosomal dominant disorder, then this would be an example of non penetrance. Penetrance (P) is usually quoted as a percentage, e.g., 80%, or as a proportion of 1, e.g., 0.8. This would imply that 80% of individuals with the gene

18

Table 2.1. Examples of Disorders That
Show Reduced Penetrance

Hereditary pancreatitis
Hereditary spastic paraplegia
Hypertrophic obstructive cardiomyopathy
Li Fraumeni syndrome
Long QT syndrome
Otosclerosis
Retinoblastoma
Tuberous sclerosis

---

will express it in some way, whereas the remaining 20% of heterozygotes will be totally unaffected. One particular issue that can generate some very difficult risk calculations is that of age-dependent penetrance. This is shown by many disorders presenting in adult life and is considered separately in Section 2.2.

In contrast to penetrance, *expressivity* (or *expression*) relates to the extent to which a disorder is manifest, so that a condition showing variable expressivity may be mild in one individual but severe in another. One potentially helpful way of grasping the distinction between penetrance and expressivity is to remember that penetrance is an all-or-none statistical parameter relating to a population, whereas expressivity is a descriptive term relating to each individual. Complete absence of expression would constitute an example of nonpenetrance. Variable expressivity is discussed further in Section 2.3.

For conditions showing reduced penetrance (Table 2.1), risks can be calculated in the following way if a value for P can be obtained from the literature. Well-known examples include otosclerosis ($P = 0.5$) and retinoblastoma ($P = 0.8–0.9$). Reduced penetrance in retinoblastoma can be explained by the absence of a second mutational event (*hit*) in a dividing retinal cell. Alternative explanations include mutations that have a mild effect on gene function (Bremner et al., 1997) and mosaicism (Chapter 6)

Example 1

Individual II1 in Figure 2.1 has a disorder showing autosomal dominant inheritance with penetrance equal to 0.8. The probability that II1 will inherit the gene *and* be affected can be calculated simply as $1/2 \times P = 0.4$.

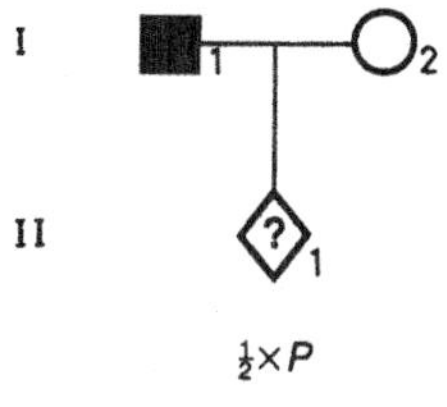

Figure 2.1. If an autosomal dominant disorder shows reduced penetrance (P), then the risk to each child of an affected individual equals $1/2 \times P$.

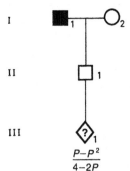

Figure 2.2. Risk to the child of an unaffected offspring of an individual with an autosomal dominant disorder showing reduced penetrance.

Example 2

Individual II1 in Figure 2.2, who is entirely normal, wishes to know of possible risks to his children. This is approached using a Bayesian calculation, as shown in Table 2.2.

The posterior probability that II1 is heterozygous, taking into account the fact that he is clinically unaffected, is

$$\frac{1/2(1-P)}{1/2(1-P)+1/2} = \frac{1-P}{2-P}$$

Thus, the probability that III1 will be clinically affected equals his father's posterior probability of heterozygosity times 1/2 (the probability that III1 will inherit a mutant allele) times P (the probability that III1 will be affected if the mutant allele is inherited), i.e.,

$$\frac{1-P}{2-P} \times \frac{1}{2} \times P = \frac{P-P^2}{4-2P}$$

Risks for III1 have been calculated for various values of P (Pauli and Motulsky, 1981) and are indicated in Table 2.3, which shows that the maximum risk is 0.086 (approximately 1 in 12) at a value of $P=0.6$. Essentially, this risk is made up of two opposing trends. At low values of P, there is a relatively high probability that III1 will be heterozygous, but given the low penetrance, it is unlikely that he or she will be clinically affected. At high values of P, it becomes much less probable that

Table 2.2.

Probability	II1 Heterozygous	II1 Not Heterozygous
Prior	$\frac{1}{2}$	$\frac{1}{2}$
Conditional Clinically normal	$1-P$	1
Joint	$\frac{1}{2}(1-P)$	$\frac{1}{2}$

Table 2.3.

1 Penetrance (P)	2 Probability That II1 Is Heterozygous $1 - P/2 - P$	3 Probability That III1 Will Be Heterozygous $1 - P/2 - P \times 1/2$	4 Probability That III1 Will Be Affected $P - P^2/4 - 2P$
0.1	0.474	0.237	0.024
0.2	0.444	0.222	0.044
0.3	0.412	0.206	0.062
0.4	0.375	0.188	0.075
0.5	0.333	0.167	0.083
0.6	0.286	0.143	0.086
0.7	0.231	0.116	0.081
0.8	0.167	0.084	0.067
0.9	0.091	0.046	0.041

See Example 2 (Fig. 2.2) In column 4 values are given for the probability that an affected child will be born to a clinically normal parent who is at a 50% prior risk of being heterozygous.

Source: Reproduced in part from Pauli and Motulsky (1981) with permission from the BMJ Publishing Group.

III1 is heterozygous, but in that event the high penetrance makes it likely that III1 will be affected.

Key Point 1

The maximum risk of an individual being affected, whose grandparent has an auto-somal dominant disorder showing reduced penetrance and whose intervening parent is unaffected, equals 0.086 or approximately 1 in 12.

Example 3

This is an extension of Example 2. Now II1 in Figure 2.3 in has n unaffected children and wishes to know the probability that his next child (III $n + 1$) will be affected. These n unaffected children further reduce the probability that II1 is heterozygous. The precise reduction in risk for III $n + 1$ can be calculated using a Bayesian cal-culation, as shown in Table 2.4. Those wishing to bypass this laborious procedure can simply refer directly to Table 2.5.

The posterior probability that II1 is heterozygous, taking into account that he is clinically unaffected and has n unaffected children, is

$$\frac{\frac{(1-P)}{(2-P)}\left(1 - \frac{P}{2}\right)^n}{\frac{(1-P)}{(2-P)}\left(1 - \frac{P}{2}\right)^n + \frac{1}{2-P}} = \frac{(1 - P)\left(1 - \frac{P}{2}\right)^n}{(1 - P)\left(1 - \frac{P}{2}\right)^n + 1}$$

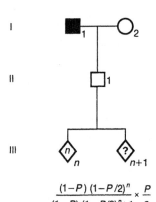

$$\frac{(1-P)\,(1-P/2)^n}{(1-P)\,(1-P/2)^{n}+1} \times \frac{P}{2}$$

Figure 2.3. Risk to the grandchild of an individual with an autosomal dominant disorder showing reduced penetrance given that II1 is unaffected and already has n unaffected children.

Table 2.4.

Probability	II1 Heterozygous	II1 Not Heterozygous
Prior	$(1-P)/(2-P)$	$\frac{1}{2}\Big/\left(\frac{1}{2}+\frac{1}{2}(1-P)\right)=(1/2-P)$
Conditional		
n normal children	$\left[\frac{1}{2}+\frac{1}{2}(1-P)\right]^n=(1-P/2)^n$	1
Joint	$((1-P)/(2-P))(1-P/2)^n$	$1/(2-P)$

Table 2.5. Maximum Risk of Being Clinically Affected for III$n+1$ in Figure 2.3 (Example 3) Given That He/She Already Has n Normal Siblings

Number of Normal Sibs (n)	Maximum Risk of Being Clinically Affected	Approximate Value of P for Maximum Risk
0	0.086	0.6
1	0.068	0.5
2	0.056	0.4
3	0.047	0.4
4	0.041	0.3
5	0.036	0.3
6	0.031	0.3
7	0.028	0.2
8	0.026	0.2
9	0.024	0.2
10	0.022	0.2

Source: From Aylsworth and Kirkman (1979) with permission of the March of Dimes Birth Defects Foundation.

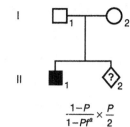

Figure 2.4. Risk to the sibling of an isolated case of an auto-somal dominant disorder showing reduced penetrance.

$$\frac{1-P}{1-Pf^a} \times \frac{P}{2}$$

The probability that III$n + 1$ will be clinically affected is the posterior probability of heterozygosity for II1 times 1/2 times P. Maximum risks, given that II1 already has n normal offspring, are given in Table 2.5. The approach to the derivation of these figures has been discussed at length by Aylsworth and Kirkman (1979).

Example 4

In this example, II1 in Figure 2.4 has an autosomal dominant condition and is an isolated case. So, in assessing the risk for II2, the critical issue is whether the disorder in II1 has arisen as a new mutation or whether I1 or I2 is an example of nonpenetrance. The important alternative explanation of parental germline mosaicism is considered in Chapter 6 (p. 120). As in previous examples, the problem is approached using a Bayesian calculation.

The prior probability that either I1 or I2 is heterozygous equals the probability that I1 is heterozygous and I2 is not, i.e., $2pq \times (1 - 2pq)$, plus the probability that I2 is heterozygous and I1 is not, i.e., $2pq \times (1 - 2pq)$. Note that it is conventional to denote the gene frequencies of the normal (= wild) and abnormal (= mutant) alleles as p and q, respectively. The derivation of $2pq$ is explained in the section on Hardy-Weinberg equilibrium in Chapter 3. Since $1 - 2pq$ will be very close to 1, the prior probability that either I1 or I2 is heterozygous can reasonably be approximated to $4pq$. The prior probability that both I1 and I2 are heterozygous $= (2pq)^2$, a very unlikely event that can be ignored.

The calculation now proceeds as shown in Table 2.6.

Table 2.6.

Probability	One Parent Heterozygous	Neither Parent Heterozygous
Prior	$4pq$	$1 - 4pq = 1$
Conditional		
Parents clinically normal	$1 - P$	1
One affected child	$\frac{1}{2}P$	$2\mu P$
Joint	$4pq(1 - P)(P/2)$	$2\mu P$

The posterior probability $P(H)$ that one parent is an example of nonpenetrance can be stated as

$$P(H) = \frac{4pq(1 - P)P/2}{4pq(1 - P)P/2 + 2\mu P} \tag{1}$$

In practice, the mutation rate (μ) is usually not known. To get around this problem, the equation originally derived by Haldane (1949) is used, i.e.,

$$\mu = \frac{I}{2}(1 - f)$$

where

$$\mu = \text{mutation rate}$$
$$I = \text{incidence of the disorder}$$
$$f = \text{fitness of heterozygotes}$$

The derivation of this equation assumes that the incidence of the disorder does not change from generation to generation, so that the number of cases arising from new mutations equals the number lost as a result of selection against affected individuals.

For the purpose of the calculation, Haldane's formula has to be modified in two ways. First, I is substituted for by $2pq$ since the incidence of the disease will equal the incidence of heterozygotes. This may be more readily understood by consulting the section on Hardy-Weinberg equilibrium in Chapter 3. The second change involves f, the fitness of all heterozygotes, which will be a function of the fitness of affected heterozygotes (f^a) and nonpenetrant heterozygotes (f^n), the latter value equalling 1. Thus, $f = Pf^a + 1 - P$.

Taking into account these two changes in Haldane's formula, equation (1) now becomes

$$P(H) = \frac{4pq(1 - P)P/2}{4pq(1 - P)P/2 + 2pq[1 - (Pf^a + 1 - P)]P}$$

which conveniently reduces by simple algebra to

$$P(H) = \frac{1 - P}{1 - Pf^a}$$

and the probability that II2 in Figure 2.4 will be both heterozygous and affected will be

$$\frac{1 - P}{1 - Pf^a} \times \frac{P}{2}$$

Therefore, if reasonable estimates for penetrance and fitness are available, the posterior probability of heterozygosity in one parent and the risk that a future child will be clinically affected can be calculated. Various approaches to the derivation of these formulae have been described (Emery, 1986; Friedman, 1985), and examples of risks to siblings of an isolated case given different values of penetrance and fitness are given in Table 2.7. It is notable that if the fitness of affected

Table 2.7. Recurrence Risks for a Sibling of an Isolated Case of a Disorder Showing Autosomal Dominant Inheritance with Reduced Penetrance and Fitness (n = number of healthy siblings)

									Fitness							
	0.3				0.5				0.7				0.9			
	n				n				n				n			
Penetrance	0	1	2	3	0	1	2	3	0	1	2	3	0	1	2	3
0.6	0.146	0.12	0.095	0.074	0.171	0.145	0.119	0.094	0.207	0.183	0.156	0.130	0.261	0.247	0.23	0.209
0.7	0.133	0.1	0.072	0.05	0.162	0.125	0.093	0.067	0.206	0.169	0.132	0.099	0.284	0.258	0.225	0.189
0.8	0.105	0.071	0.046	0.029	0.133	0.086	0.061	0.039	0.182	0.133	0.092	0.061	0.286	0.24	0.189	0.14
0.9	0.070	0.036	0.021	0.012	0.082	0.049	0.028	0.016	0.122	0.076	0.045	0.026	0.237	0.171	0.113	0.07

Key Point 2

When unaffected parents have a child with an autosomal dominant disorder that shows reduced penetrance, a sibling recurrence risk can be calculated, or taken from Table 2.7, if estimates for the disease penetrance and fitness can be obtained.

---

heterozygotes equals 1, then the probability that one of the parents is also heterozygous also equals 1. Thus, the risk to the next sibling equals $P/2$. This is a consequence of the previous assumption that the disorder shows mutation–selection equilibrium, implying that if there is no selection against heterozygotes, then there will be no cases resulting from new mutations.

There are several important points to keep in mind when using this approach. First, this exercise is applicable only after the family has been thoroughly investigated and the counselor is satisfied that no one else in the family shows any signs of the relevant disorder. Second, accurate figures for penetrance and fitness are not always easy to find, so values for these parameters may have to be estimated. Finally, the availability of specific mutation analysis may make it possible to establish that neither parent carries the mutation found in the affected child, so that the possibility of nonpenetrance can be excluded.

Example 5

This example is very similar to the situation discussed in Example 4, but the risk to a future child is now modified by the existence of n healthy siblings. The greater the number of healthy siblings, the more likely it is that the disease in the isolated case is the result of a new mutation as opposed to inheritance from a nonpenetrant heterozygous parent. Calculation of the precise risk to $\text{II}n + 2$ in Figure 2.5 proceeds as shown in Table 2.8.

By applying this Bayesian calculation, as in Example 4, it can be shown that the probability that $\text{II}\,n + 2$ in Figure 2.5 will be both heterozygous and affected equals

$$\frac{(1 - P)(1 - P/2)^n}{(1 - P)(1 - P/2)^n + P(1 - f^a)} \times \frac{P}{2}$$

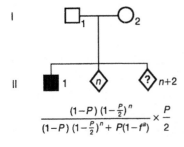

$$\frac{(1-P)(1-\frac{P}{2})^n}{(1-P)(1-\frac{P}{2})^n + P(1-f^a)} \times \frac{P}{2}$$

Figure 2.5. Risk to the sibling of an isolated case of an autosomal dominant disorder showing reduced penetrance given that there are n healthy siblings.

Table 2.8.

Probability	One Parent Heterozygous	Neither Parent Heterozygous
Prior	$4pq$	1
Conditional		
Parents clinically normal	$1 - P$	1
One affected child	$\frac{1}{2}P$	$2\mu P$
n unaffected children	$\left[\frac{1}{2} + \frac{1}{2}(1 - P)\right]^{n} = (1 - (P/2))^{n}$	1
Joint	$4pq(1 - P)(P/2)(1 - (P/2))^{n}$	$2\mu P$

Risks of recurrence for different values of fitness and penetrance given for 0–3 healthy siblings are presented in Table 2.7. For a condition such as hereditary retinoblastoma, in which penetrance is equal to approximately 0.9 and fitness is probably equal to approximately 0.5 (allowing for reduced fitness because of morbidity and mortality associated with primary and secondary tumors), it is apparent from Table 2.7 that the risk of recurrence will vary from approximately 8% if there are no unaffected siblings to just over 1% if there are three unaffected siblings. These figures are comparable to those that have been observed in practice, as discussed further in the section on germline mosaicism in Chapter 6 (p. 124).

2.2 Disorders with Late Onset (Age-Dependent Penetrance)

Many conditions showing autosomal dominant inheritance are characterized by onset at variable age in adult life. Increasingly specific mutation testing or linkage analysis can be used for predictive purposes, but sometimes molecular testing is not available or relevant key individuals may refuse to provide samples. In these situations, a simple calculation can be carried out to modify an individual's prior risk based on his or her age. A useful example for illustrative purposes is Huntington disease, for which life table data can be used to provide estimates of the probability that an individual at prior risk of 50% is heterozygous if clinically unaffected at a particular age (Table 2.9). Example 6 illustrates how these risks have been derived. Example 7 shows how unaffected grandchildren can also be taken into account.

Example 6

A healthy 60-year-old man (II1 in Fig. 2.6) presents with a history of his father having had Huntington disease. II1 must therefore have commenced life at a 50% risk of inheriting a Huntington disease mutation. This prior probability of 50% (= 0.5) can be modified using a Bayesian calculation, as shown in Table 2.10. The conditional probability of 0.25 for II1 being heterozygous is derived from Table 2.9,

Table 2.9. Approximate Risks at Different Ages for Clinically Unaffected Individuals Who Are at 50% Risk of Huntington Disease (See Example 6)

Age in Years	Probability of Detectable Gene Expression	Probability of Heterozygosity If Clinically Unaffected
20	0.02	0.49
25	0.05	0.48
30	0.1	0.47
35	0.2	0.44
40	0.3	0.41
45	0.35	0.39
50	0.5	0.33
55	0.65	0.26
60	0.75	0.20
65	0.85	0.13
70	0.95	0.05

Source: Data adapted from Harper and Newcombe (1992) with permission from the BMJ Publishing Group.

which indicates that 75% of heterozygotes are affected by age 60 years. Thus, from Table 2.10, it can be calculated that the probability that II1 is heterozygous equals $0.125/(0.125 + 0.5)$, which equals 0.2, a considerable decrease from his prior probability of 0.5.

Example 7

Figure 2.6 shows that II1 has one son (III1) and one daughter (III2) who are also in good health. This information can be utilized to reduce the prior probability of 0.5 even further, as shown in Table 2.11.

This yields a posterior probability of $0.095625/0.595625 = 0.16$ that II1 has inherited the Huntington disease gene. Therefore, information provided by III1 and III2 has resulted in a further reduction of risk for II1 from 0.2 (1 in 5) to 0.16 (approximately 1 in 6).

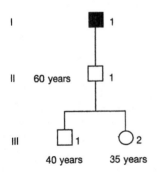

I

II   60 years

III

40 years   35 years

Figure 2.6. I1 has an autosomal dominant disorder showing variable age of onset in adult life. The approach to estimating risks for II1, III1, and III2 is discussed in the text.

Table 2.10.

Probability	II1 Is Heterozygous	II1 Is Homozygous Normal
Prior	0.5	0.5
Conditional		
Healthy at age 60 years	0.25	1
Joint	0.125	0.5

Table 2.11.

Probability	II1 Is Heterozygous	II1 Is Homozygous Normal
Prior	0.5	0.5
Conditional		
(1) II1 age 60 years	0.25	1
(2) III1 age 40 years	$0.5 + (0.5 \times 0.7) = 0.85$	1
(3) III2 age 35 years	$0.5 + (0.5 \times 0.8) = 0.90$	1
Joint	0.095625	0.5

Table 2.12.

Probability	II1 Is Heterozygous	II1 Is Homozygous Normal
Prior	0.5	0.5
Conditional		
(1) II1 age 60 years	0.25	1
(2) III1 age 40 years	0.85	1
Joint	0.10625	0.5

Table 2.13.

Probability	III2 Is Heterozygous	III2 Is Homozygous Normal
Prior	0.0875	0.9125
Conditional		
III2 age 35 years	0.8	1
Joint	0.07	0.9125

It is important to note that posterior risks for III1 and III2 should not be calculated using a prior risk for each of $0.16 \times 1/2$, as information provided by these individuals has already been used in deriving this posterior probability of 0.16 for II1. If III2 wishes to know the probability that she is heterozygous, the calculation is as shown in Tables 2.12 and 2.13.

Table 2.12 yields a provisional posterior probability of heterozygosity for II1 of $0.10625/0.60625 = 0.175$. The prior probability for III2 can now be calculated by halving this value of 0.175 and proceeding as shown in Table 2.13. The posterior probability that III2 has inherited Huntington disease equals $0.07/0.9825$, which equals approximately 0.07 or 7%.

Key Point 3

When counseling for an autosomal dominant disorder showing variable age of onset, genetic risks can be modified using Bayes' theorem by utilizing information from an age-of-onset table. A conditional probability can be obtained by asking the key question, "What is the probability that the consultand would be clinically unaffected at his/her age if he/she has inherited the mutant allele?"

2.3 Variable Expression

Many autosomal dominant disorders show quite striking variation in severity not only between families but also within them, so that a mildly affected parent may have a severely affected child or vice versa. Neurofibromatosis type 1 is an example of a relatively common autosomal dominant disorder in which affected family members can show markedly different degrees of severity in both the major diagnostic features and the development of complications. Discordance between MZ twin pairs is less marked than that between other relatives, indicating that both environmental factors and other genes are implicated (Easton et al., 1993).

Often a mildly affected parent will not be too concerned about the possibility of having an equally mildly affected child but will be very anxious that a child could be severely affected. Figures for the incidence of severe complications can sometimes be obtained from comprehensive studies and reviews, although there is a danger that the risk of serious problems will have been overestimated because of biased ascertainment, i.e., those with serious complications are much more likely to come to medical attention.

Incidence figures for potentially serious complications in some of the more common autosomal dominant disorders are given in Table 2.14. These can be used to modify the 50% risk applying to future children. For example, a parent with the classical mild form of osteogenesis imperfecta (type I) can reasonably be told that a future child, if affected, runs a 3% risk of being so severely disabled by fractures

Table 2.14. Examples of Serious Complications That Can Occur in Specific Autosomal Dominant Disorders

Disorder	Complication	Incidence
Facioscapulohumeral muscular dystrophy	Severe disability by age 40 years	20%
Hereditary motor and sensory neuropathy—type I	Major difficulty in walking by age 40 years	5%–10%
Multiple exostoses	Sarcoma	3%
Neurofibromatosis 1	Malignancy	3%
	Requirement for special school education	10%
Osteogenesis imperfecta—type I	Deafness	40%
	Wheelchair dependence	3%
Retinoblastoma	Osteosarcoma	18%–26%
Tuberous sclerosis	Epilepsy	60%
	Mental retardation	40%
Waardenburg syndrome	Deafness	
Type I		25%
Type II		50%

that a wheelchair will be necessary. Thus, overall, there will be a risk of $0.5 \times 3\% = 1.5\%$ that a future child will be wheelchair dependent.

Key Point 4

The risk that a child will both inherit a disorder and develop a particular serious complication can be calculated by multiplying the pedigree risk (1 in 2) by the incidence of the complication.

2.4 Parents Have Two Different Autosomal Dominant Disorders

Occasionally, a family is encountered in which two disorders are segregating. Parents may wish to know the likelihood that a child could inherit both, one, or none of these conditions. Two possible situations are considered.

Each Parent Has a Different Disorder

A formal approach to estimating the risks for children is shown in the form of a Punnett's square in Figure 2.7. It can be seen that there are 16 possible combinations of parental alleles. The risks for children are as might be expected intuitively, i.e., 1 in 4 for both disorders, 1 in 4 for the maternal disorder only, 1 in 4 for the paternal

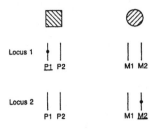

Locus 1 (P1 = mutant allele)

	P1 M1	P1 M2	P2 M1	P2 M2
	P1 M1	P1 M2	P2 M1	P2 M2
P1 M1	P1 M1	P1 M1	P1 M1	P1 M1
	P1 M1	P1 M2	P2 M1	P2 M2
P1 M2	P1 M2	P1 M2	P1 M2	P1 M2
	P1 M1	P1 M2	P2 M1	P2 M2
P2 M1	P2 M1	P2 M1	P2 M1	P2 M1
	P1 M1	P1 M2	P2 M1	P2 M2
P2 M2	P2 M2	P2 M2	P2 M2	P2 M2

Locus 2 (M2 = mutant allele)

Figure 2.7. Risks for offspring of parents each of whom has a different autosomal dominant disorder. On average 1 in 4 will have both, 1 in 4 the paternal disorder, 1 in 4 the maternal disorder, and 1 in 4 neither.

disorder only, and 1 in 4 for neither disorder. These risks can be derived much more simply by multiplying 1/2 by 1/2 for each outcome, e.g., the risk of inheriting the paternal disorder (1/2) but not the maternal disorder (1/2) equals 1/4.

Key Point 5

When parents each have a different autosomal dominant disorder or when one parent has such disorders, the chances that a child will inherit both, one, or neither disorder are 1 in 4, 1 in 2, and 1 in 4, respectively.

One Parent Has Two Disorders

The approach to this situation is outlined in Figure 2.8. The risks are essentially the same as in the previous situation but with one important proviso. If the loci of the two disorders are linked (i.e., close together on the same chromosome so that separation by recombination at meiosis is unlikely), then the two disorders will not segregate independently. Risks to offspring will depend on whether the two mutant alleles are on the same chromosome (*in coupling*) or on opposite chromosomes (*in repulsion*). In the absence of a family history, it may not be possible to know whether the disorders are in coupling or in repulsion. However, if the patient

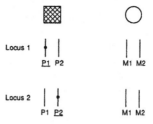

Locus 1 (P1 = mutant allele)

	P1 M1	P1 M2	P2 M1	P2 M2
Locus 2 (P2 = mutant allele)	P1 M1	P1 M2	P2 M1	P2 M2
P1 M1	P1 M1	P1 M1	P1 M1	P1 M1
	P1 M1	P1 M2	P2 M1	P2 M2
P1 M2	P1 M2	P1 M2	P1 M2	P1 M2
	P1 M1	P1 M2	P2 M1	P2 M2
P2 M1	P2 M1	P2 M1	P2 M1	P2 M1
	P1 M1	P1 M2	P2 M1	P2 M2
P2 M2	P2 M2	P2 M2	P2 M2	P2 M2

Figure 2.8. Risks for offspring of parents, one of whom has two autosomal dominant disorders. On average, 1 in 4 will have both, 1 in 2 will have one, and 1 in 4 will have neither.

inherited both conditions from the same parent, then clearly the mutant alleles will be in coupling; if from different parents, then they will be in repulsion.

If the mutant alleles are very tightly linked on the same chromosome, then the risk to each child will be 50% for inheriting both disorders and 50% for inheriting neither. If the two mutant alleles are on opposite chromosomes, then on average 50% of the children will inherit one disorder and the remaining 50% will inherit the other disorder.

The likelihood of recombination between two loci is known as the *recombination fraction* (θ) (p. 94). If a value of 5% (= 0.05) is assumed, then risks can be modified as indicated in Figure 2.9. If the mutant alleles are in coupling (on the same chromosome), then risks for offspring will be:

47.5% for both diseases

47.5% for neither disease

2.5% for one disease only

2.5% for the other disease only.

If the mutant alleles are in repulsion (on opposite chromosomes), then risks for offspring will be:

2.5% for both diseases

47.5% for one disease only

47.5% for the other disease only

2.5% for neither disease.

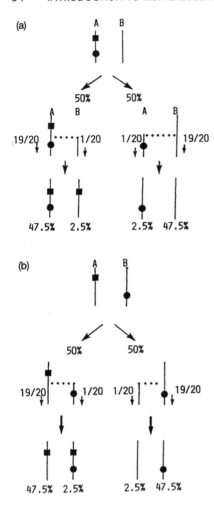

Figure 2.9. Risks for offspring of parents, one of whom has two linked autosomal dominant disorders with a recombination fraction of 5%.

The concept of genetic linkage and its application in risk calculation are considered at much greater length in Chapter 5.

2.5 Parents Have the Same Autosomal Dominant Disorder

When two individuals with the same autosomal dominant disorder have a child, the outcome will be as shown in Figure 2.10. This indicates that there will be a probability of 1 in 4 that a child will inherit two normal alleles, 1 in 2 that a child will inherit one normal and one mutant allele, and 1 in 4 that a child will inherit two mutant alleles.

Thus, on average, three out of four offspring will inherit at least one mutant allele. According to the classical definition of dominance, a single copy of a mutant

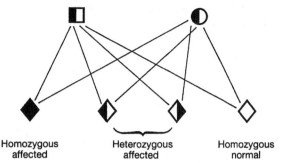

Figure 2.10. Risks for offspring of parents, both of whom have the same autosomal dominant disorder.

Homozygous affected   Heterozygous affected   Homozygous normal

allele results in the same clinical problems as in the mutant homozygote. In practice, as has been pointed out by Pauli (1983) and Zlotogora (1997), this is not usually so. For most autosomal dominant disorders, a double dose of the mutant allele results in much more severe clinical expression of the disease than is usually seen in a heterozygote.

Examples of the clinical effects of homozygosity for various autosomal dominant disorders are given in Table 2.15. It is apparent that for most of these conditions the effects are very severe. Curiously, homozygotes for Huntington disease, Creutzfeld-Jakob disease, and myotonic dystrophy are no more severely affected than heterozygotes. These three disorders are thought to be caused by gain-of-function mutations, in contrast to several of the other disorders listed in Table 2.15, such as aniridia and Waardenburg syndrome, which are caused by loss-of-function (*haploinsufficiency*) mutations. However, there is no clear relationship between the type of mutation and its outcome in heterozygotes, compared to homozygotes, so that at present the explanation for why some disorders show true dominance in the classical sense remains unknown.

Key Point 6

There is 1 chance in 4 that a child born to parents who both have the same autosomal dominant disorder will inherit both mutant alleles and therefore will be homozygous. In most disorders the homozygote is much more severely affected than the heterozygote.

2.6 Affected Siblings Born to Unaffected Parents

Occasionally, a family is encountered in which entirely healthy parents have had two or more children with the same autosomal dominant disorder. Such a family presents a very difficult counseling problem. In attempting to provide a recurrence risk, several possible explanations have to be considered:

Table 2.15. Clinical Outcome of Homozygosity in Autosomal Dominant Disorders

Disorder	Outcome
Achondroplasia	Severe skeletal dysplasia with early lethality
Aniridia	Absence of facial structures
Creutzfeld-Jakob disease	No difference from heterozygote
Dentatorubral-pallidoluysian atrophy	Earlier onset and more severe
Dyschondrosteosis	Langer type of mesomelic dysplasia, i.e., severe limb shortening
Elliptocytosis	Severe anemia, possibly lethal in early infancy
Familial hypercholesterolemia	Coronary artery disease by second to third decade
Hereditary hemorrhagic telangiectasia	Stillborn with visceral angiomatous malformations
Hereditary motor and sensory neuropathy (type I)	Early onset of severe muscle weakness and wasting
Huntington disease	No difference from heterozygote
Marfan syndrome	Severe congenital involvement with death in early infancy
Myotonic dystrophy	No difference from heterozygote
Spinocerebellar ataxia (type 3)	Early onset and more rapid progression
Synpolydactyly	Severe hand and foot abnormalities
Waardenburg syndrome	Partial albinism and limb defects
Von Willebrand disease	Early onset and more severe bleeding diathesis

1. The disorder may show reduced penetrance, with one of the parents being a nonpenetrant heterozygote.
2. The original mutation may have occurred in an early germline mitotic division in one of the parents, who is therefore said to show *germline mosaicism.*
3. One of the parents may carry the gene as a *premutation,* i.e., the mutation exists in a clinically silent, unstable form that can undergo a further change in meiosis resulting in a full pathogenic mutation. This is often referred to as *anticipation.*
4. Two independent new mutations could have occurred in the gametes that resulted in the conception of the two affected siblings.
5. Paternity may not be as claimed.
6. The disorder may show genetic heterogeneity with a rare autosomal recessive form accounting for the affected siblings.

Distinguishing between these various possibilities can be extremely difficult. Sometimes consideration of the disorder in question may help indicate which of these underlying mechanisms is the most likely. For example, some disorders are known to show reduced penetrance (Table 2.1). If this is thought to be the most likely mechanism, then it is reasonable to quote a recurrence risk of $1/2 \times P$, where P equals penetrance, as discussed previously (p. 19).

For other conditions, such as facioscapulohumeral muscular dystrophy and the severe forms of osteogenesis imperfecta, germline mosaicism is a more probable explanation. In these situations, counseling is often based on observed "empiric" risks to future siblings (p. 124). Alternatively, theoretical risks have been derived

Table 2.16. Disorders That Show Anticipation

Disorder	Inheritance	Transmission
Dentatorubral-pallidoluysian atrophy	AD	Paternal
Fragile X syndrome	X-linked	Maternal
Huntington disease	AD	Paternal
Myotonic dystrophy	AD	Maternal
Spinocerebellar ataxia type 1	AD	Paternal
Spinocerebellar ataxia type 3 (Machado-Joseph disease)	AD	Paternal
Spinocerebellar ataxia type 7	AD	Paternal

AD, autosomal dominant.

based on the structure of the sibship and various estimates of the number of cell divisions in germline development (Chapter 6). The derivation of these risks involves several important assumptions, and these recurrence risks should be modified downward if the sibship contains unaffected children (p. 126).

Until recently the third explanation, i.e., a premutation, was largely hypothetical, being based on studies in *Drosophila*. However, this type of mutation is now widely recognized as occurring in several autosomal dominant disorders, many of which present with progressive neurological disability in adult life, as well as in the Fragile X syndrome, which shows a modified form of X-linked inheritance (Table 2.16). Consequently, this third possible explanation of a unique type of parental "premutation" should be considered carefully, particularly if the disorder in question shows progressive neurological involvement. This subject is considered at greater length in the next section.

Key Point 7

When unaffected parents have two children with the same autosomal dominant disorder, possible explanations include reduced penetrance, germline mosaicism, and a premutation. Consideration of the disorder in question will often indicate which is the most likely explanation.

It is worth emphasizing that consideration of the most plausible underlying mechanism has implications not only for the sibling recurrence risk but also for members of future generations. This can be illustrated by considering individual II3 in Figure 2.11. If the disorder affecting siblings II1 and II2 has resulted from parental germline mosaicism for a fully penetrant gene, then II3, who is unaffected, can be reassured that the risk to his future offspring is negligible. However, if one of the parents, I1 or I2, is an example of nonpenetrance or a carrier of a premutation, then II3 could also be an unaffected heterozygote and therefore be at risk of having affected children.

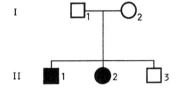

Figure 2.11. II1 and II2 have the same autosomal dominant disorder. Estimation of the risk for II3 is discussed in the text.

2.7 Anticipation

Anticipation refers to the phenomenon whereby a small number of genetic disorders, most of which show autosomal dominant inheritance and are caused by unstable triplet repeat mutations, demonstrate increasing severity and/or earlier age of onset in succeeding generations (Table 2.16). This is particularly relevant for Huntington disease, myotonic dystrophy, and the X-linked Fragile X syndrome. When counseling families in which one of these disorders is segregating, it is common to be asked to predict the degree of severity or age of onset in mutation carriers in either the present or the next generation. These requests are entirely reasonable but, unfortunately, cannot always be answered with confidence. However, experience with these conditions has accumulated to the extent that it is now sometimes possible to provide an indication of disease severity based on knowledge of the transmitting parent and analysis of the mutation in relevant family members. This is illustrated by consideration of recent observations in Huntington disease.

Huntington disease is caused by an expanded unstable CAG triplet repeat in the Huntingtin gene on chromosome 4. There is a well-established inverse relationship between the length of the triplet repeat and the age of onset, and this relationship is now sufficiently robust to allow individual risk prediction. Based on the analysis of almost 3000 individuals from Huntington disease families, an international collaborative group has derived population estimates of the mean age of onset for CAG repeat lengths from 36 to 60 (Langbehn et al., 2004). The large size of this

---

Key Point 8

Disorders that show anticipation include Huntington disease in paternal transmission and both the Fragile X syndrome and myotonic dystrophy in maternal transmission. This possibility should be included in a discussion of genetic risks. Figures are now becoming available that enable prediction of age of onset and/or severity based on the size of the triplet repeat.

---

sample has allowed narrow confidence intervals to be defined (Fig. 2.12). Figures have also been derived for the probability that an individual with an expansion mutation will develop the condition at various 5-year intervals (Table 2.17).

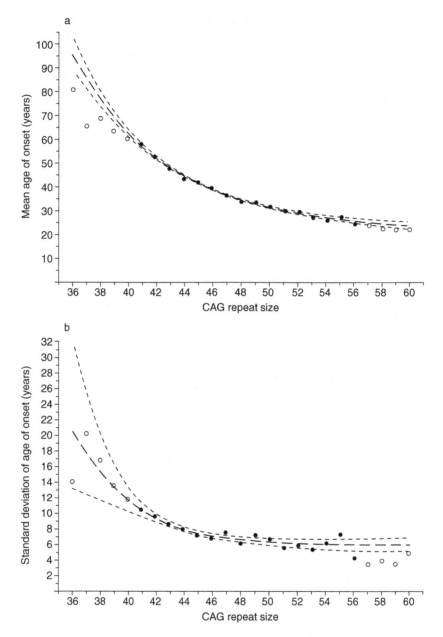

Figure 2.12. Estimates of the mean age of onset with 95% confidence intervals (a) and standard deviation of the age of onset (b) for CAG repeat lengths in Huntington disease. Solid symbols and lines indicate the range of data used to fit exponential curves. Open symbols and long dashed lines indicate CAG lengths for which the predictions were extrapolated. (Reproduced with permission of the publishers, Blackwell Munksgaard, from Langbeehn et al., 2004. A new model for prediction of the age of onset and penetrance for Huntington's disease based on CAG length. Clinical Genetics, 65, 267–277.)

Table 2.17. Probability of Onset of Huntington Disease at 5-Year Intervals for a 40-Year-Old Individual Based on CAG Repeat Size

CAG Repeat Size	Conditional Probability (95% CI) of Onset for an Individual 40* Years by Age						
	45 Years	50 Years	55 Years	60 Years	65 Years	70 Years	75 Years
36	<0.01 (0–0.02)	0.01 (0–0.05)	0.02 (0–0.08)	0.04 (0.01–0.12)	0.06 (0.02–0.16)	0.09 (0.03–0.22)	0.14 (0.06–0.28)
37	0.01 (0–0.02)	0.02 (0.01–0.05)	0.03 (0.01–0.09)	0.06 (0.03–0.14)	0.10 (0.05–0.20)	0.17 (0.09–0.28)	0.25 (0.16–0.37)
38	0.01 (0–0.03)	0.03 (0.01–0.06)	0.06 (0.03–0.11)	0.11 (0.07–0.19)	0.19 (0.13–0.28)	0.31 (0.23–0.40)	0.45 (0.35–0.54)
39	0.02 (0.01–0.03)	0.05 (0.03–0.08)	0.11 (0.08–0.16)	0.21 (0.16–0.28)	0.35 (0.29–0.43)	0.52 (0.45–0.60)	0.68 (0.60–0.76)
40	0.03 (0.02–0.05)	0.10 (0.08–0.13)	0.21 (0.18–0.26)	0.38 (0.33–0.43)	0.58 (0.52–0.63)	0.75 (0.69–0.80)	0.87 (0.82–0.90)
41	0.06 (0.05–0.08)	0.19 (0.17–0.21)	0.38 (0.35–0.42)	0.60 (0.57–0.64)	0.79 (0.75–0.82)	0.90 (0.87–0.92)	0.95 (0.94–0.97)
42	0.12 (0.11–0.13)	0.34 (0.32–0.36)	0.59 (0.57–0.62)	0.80 (0.78–0.82)	0.91 (0.90–0.93)	0.96 (0.96–0.97)	0.99 (0.98–0.99)
43	0.22 (0.21–0.24)	0.53 (0.51–0.55)	0.78 (0.76–0.80)	0.91 (0.90–0.92)	0.97 (0.96–0.97)	0.99 (0.96–0.97)	>0.99 (>0.99->0.99)
44	0.36 (0.34–0.38)	0.70 (0.67–0.72)	0.89 (0.87–0.90)	0.96 (0.95–0.97)	0.99 (0.98–0.99)	>0.99 (>0.99->0.99)	>0.99 (>0.99->0.99)
45	0.50 (0.47–0.52)	0.81 (0.79–0.83)	0.94 (0.93–0.95)	0.98 (0.98–0.99)	>0.99 (>0.99->0.99)	>0.99 (>0.99->0.99)	>0.99 (>0.99->0.99)
46	0.60 (0.58–0.63)	0.87 (0.86–0.89)	0.96 (0.96–0.97)	>0.99 (>0.99->0.99)	>0.99 (>0.99->0.99)	>0.99 (>0.99->0.99)	>0.99 (>0.99->0.99)
47	0.67 (0.65–0.69)	0.91 (0.89–0.92)	0.98 (0.97–0.98)	>0.99 (>0.99->0.99)	>0.99 (>0.99->0.99)	>0.99 (>0.99->0.99)	>0.99 (>0.99->0.99)
48	0.71 (0.69–0.73)	0.92 (0.91–0.94)	0.98 (0.98–0.98)	>0.99 (>0.99->0.99)	>0.99 (>0.99->0.99)	>0.99 (>0.99->0.99)	>0.99 (>0.99->0.99)
49	0.74 (0.71–0.76)	0.93 (0.92–0.95)	0.98 (0.98–0.99)	>0.99 (>0.99->0.99)	>0.99 (>0.99->0.99)	>0.99 (>0.99->0.99)	>0.99 (>0.99->0.99)
50	0.75 (0.72–0.78)	0.94 (0.93–0.95)	0.99 (0.98–0.99)	>0.99 (>0.99->0.99)	>0.99 (>0.99->0.99)	>0.99 (>0.99->0.99)	>0.99 (>0.99->0.99)
51	0.76 (0.73–0.79)	0.94 (0.93–0.96)	0.99 (0.98->0.99)	>0.99 (>0.99->0.99)	>0.99 (>0.99->0.99)	>0.99 (>0.99->0.99)	>0.99 (>0.99->0.99)
52	0.77 (0.73–0.80)	0.95 (0.93–0.96)	0.99 (0.98->0.99)	>0.99 (>0.99->0.99)	>0.99 (>0.99->0.99)	>0.99 (>0.99->0.99)	>0.99 (>0.99->0.99)
53	0.77 (0.73–0.81)	0.95 (0.93–0.96)	0.99 (0.98->0.99)	>0.99 (>0.99->0.99)	>0.99 (>0.99->0.99)	>0.99 (>0.99->0.99)	>0.99 (>0.99->0.99)
54	0.77 (0.73–0.81)	0.95 (0.93–0.96)	0.99 (0.98->0.99)	>0.99 (>0.99->0.99)	>0.99 (>0.99->0.99)	>0.99 (>0.99->0.99)	>0.99 (>0.99->0.99)
55	0.78 (0.73–0.81)	0.95 (0.93–0.97)	0.99 (0.98->0.99)	>0.99 (>0.99->0.99)	>0.99 (>0.99->0.99)	>0.99 (>0.99->0.99)	>0.99 (>0.99->0.99)
56	0.78 (0.73–0.82)	0.95 (0.93–0.97)	0.99 (0.98->0.99)	>0.99 (>0.99->0.99)	>0.99 (>0.99->0.99)	>0.99 (>0.99->0.99)	>0.99 (>0.99->0.99)

*Predictions are available for other ages at http://www.cmmt.ubc.ca/hayden.

Source: Reproduced with permission of the publishers, Blackwell Munksgaard, from Langbehn et al. (2004).

Reference to these figures should enable counselors to give mutation carriers a reasonably accurate indication of their long-term prognosis.

At present, it is much more difficult to predict severity in a future generation based on knowledge of mutation size in a prospective parent. In Huntington disease, anticipation occurs almost exclusively in paternal transmission, with an average increase of 4 in the length of the triplet repeat and an 8-year decrease in the age of onset (Ranen et al., 1995). It would be reasonable to quote these figures, but with the important caveat that they represent the average of a very wide range of observations that include several examples of offspring showing later ages of onset than their affected fathers. Figures are now available for the likelihood that a premutation in a female Fragile X carrier will be transmitted as a full mutation. For repeat sizes of 55–59, 60–69, 70–79, 80–89, and 90–99 the risks are 3.7%, 5.3%, 31.1%, 57.8%, and 80.1%, respectively. For repeat sizes greater than 100 the risk is close to 100% (Nolin et al., 2003). As women have two X chromosomes, these percentage figures should be divided by 2 to obtain the probability that a carrier mother will actually transmit a full mutation to each of her children.

Further Reading

Langbehn, D.R., Brinkman, R.R., Falush, D., Paulsen, J.S., and Hayden, M.R. (2004). A new model for prediction of the age of onset and penetrance for Huntington's disease based on CAG length. *Clinical Genetics*, **65**, 267–277.

Strachan, T. and Read, A.P. (2004). *Human molecular genetics 3*. Garland Science, New York.

Vogel, F. and Motulsky, A.G. (1996). *Human genetics: Problems and approaches* (3rd ed.). Springer, Berlin.

Wilkie, A. (1994). The molecular basis of genetic dominance. *Journal of Medical Genetics*, **31**, 89–98.

Zlotogora, J. (1997). Dominance and homozygosity. *American Journal of Medical Genetics*, **68**, 412–416.

3

Autosomal Recessive Inheritance

The provision of risks to the parents of a child with an autosomal recessive disorder is generally straightforward, given that there is a probability of 1 in 4 that each future child born to the parents will be affected. For other family members, however, risk calculation can be much more complex, particularly if there is a history of consanguinity or if only limited carrier testing is available. Several such situations are considered in this chapter.

3.1 Hardy-Weinberg Equilibrium

Before discussing individual examples, it is necessary to dwell briefly on a fundamental principle that is often applied in risk calculation. Stated simply, *Hardy-Weinberg equilibrium* relates to the fact that in a large randomly mating population, in which two alleles, N and A (N = normal or wild type, A = abnormal or mutant), are segregating, the proportions of the three genotypes NN, NA (or AN), and AA remain constant and can be obtained from the binomial expression $(p + q)^2$, where p and q represent the frequencies of the normal and abnormal genes, respectively, and $p + q = 1$. Thus, if a population is in Hardy-Weinberg equilibrium, the frequencies of the different genotypes will be as indicated in Table 3.1.

Several factors can disturb this equilibrium, such as selection for or against a particular genotype, random fluctuation in a small population, migration, and new mutations. For practical counseling purposes these can usually be ignored, particularly as it is generally assumed that the introduction of new mutations for a recessive allele is balanced by the loss of mutant alleles resulting from selection against the affected homozygote.

The enormous value of this principle is that it enables the carrier frequency of an autosomal recessive disorder to be determined if the incidence of the disorder is known. For example, if a particular disease has an incidence of 1 in 10,000, then

42

Table 3.1.

Genotype	Phenotype	Frequency
NN	Normal	p^2
NA and AN	Normal (carrier)	$2pq$
AA	Affected	q^2

$q^2 = 1/10,000, q = 1/100$, and the carrier frequency equals $2 \times 99/100 \times 1/100$, which approximates to $1/50$. In general, a reasonable approximation of the carrier frequency can be obtained by doubling the square root of the disease incidence. Examples of carrier frequencies determined assuming Hardy-Weinberg equilibrium are given in Table 3.2. It should be noted that a carrier frequency estimated in this way will be an overestimate if the disease incidence has been obtained from a small population with a high proportion of consanguineous matings, as this leads to a greater incidence of homozygotes than would occur in a large randomly mating population. Values for the incidence and carrier frequency of some of the more commonly encountered autosomal recessive disorders are given in Table 3.3.

Key Point 1

An estimate of the carrier frequency ($2pq$) for an autosomal recessive disorder can be obtained by doubling the square root of the incidence of affected homozygotes (q^2).

3.2 Risk to the Offspring of a Healthy Sibling

The healthy brother or sister of an individual with a severe autosomal recessive disorder may well wish to know the likelihood that his or her own child could be

Table 3.2. Approximate Values for Gene Frequency and Carrier Frequency Derived from Disease Incidence Using the Hardy-Weinberg Equilibrium.

Incidence of Disease (q^2)	Gene Frequency (q)	Carrier Frequency ($2pq$)
1/100	1/10	2/11
1/1000	1/32	1/16
1/2000	1/45	1/23
1/5000	1/71	1/35
1/10,000	1/100	1/50
1/20,000	1/141	1/71
1/50,000	1/224	1/112
1/100,000	1/316	1/158

Table 3.3. Incidence and Carrier Frequency Values for Known
Autosomal Recessive Disorders

Incidence (q^2)	Carrier frequency ($2pq$)	Disorder
1/400	1/10	Hemochromatosis
		Sickle cell disease
		Thalassemia
1/2000	1/22	Cystic fibrosis
1/2500	1/25	α_1-Antitrypsin deficiency
1/3600	1/30	Tay-Sachs disease
1/5000	1/35	Congenital adrenal hyperplasia
		(21 hydroxylase deficiency)
1/10,000	1/50	Cystinuria
		Deafness (Connexin 26)
		Oculocutaneous albinism
		Phenylketonuria
		Spinal muscular atrophy
		(childhood forms)
1/17,000	1/65	Medium chain acyl-coA
		dehydrogenase deficiency
1/40,000	1/100	Friedreich's ataxia
1/160,000	1/200	Hurler syndrome
1/250,000	1/250	Ataxia-telangiectasia

affected. This risk is calculated by multiplying the independent probabilities that the sibling and his or her partner are carriers to determine the probability that both members of the partnership are carriers and then multiplying by 1 in 4, this being the probability that a child born to two carrier parents will be affected.

The mechanism underlying autosomal recessive inheritance is illustrated in Figure 3.1. From this it is apparent that, on average, two out of three *unaffected* siblings of an affected individual will be carriers. Thus, the healthy sibling can be assigned a probability of 2/3 for being a carrier, and not 1/2, as is easily misconceived. (The probability that a sibling of an affected individual is a carrier equals 2 in 4, i.e.,1 in 2, but the probability that an *unaffected* sibling is a carrier equals 2 in 3, as the denominator is now 3 and not 4.) The probability that this

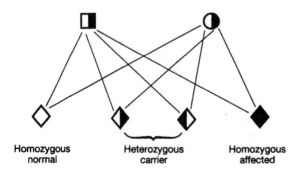

Homozygous normal   **Heterozygous carrier**   **Homozygous affected**

Figure 3.1. The mechanism underlying autosomal recessive inheritance. It can be seen that on average, two out of three of the healthy siblings of the affected individual will be carriers.

sibling's healthy and unrelated partner is a carrier is calculated using the Hardy-Weinberg equilibrium, assuming, as is likely, that an appropriate incidence figure for the disease in question can be obtained from the literature.

Key Point 2

The probability that a healthy sibling of someone with an autosomal recessive disorder is a carrier equals 2/3.

Example 1

The unaffected sister of a man with cystic fibrosis wishes to know the probability that her first child will be affected. This woman's healthy partner is not a blood relative, has no family history of cystic fibrosis, and comes from the same ethnic group as the sister, in which cystic fibrosis has an incidence of 1 in 1600. Calculation of the risk proceeds as indicated in Figure 3.2. The probability that the sister is a carrier equals 2/3. The probability that her healthy partner (II3) is a carrier equals the frequency of carriers in the general population, i.e., approximately $2\sqrt{1/1600}$, which equals 1 in 20. The probability that their first child will be affected equals the product of the probabilities of these two independent events multiplied by 1 in 4, the chance that they will both pass on the gene (i.e., have an affected child) if they are carriers. This therefore gives a risk of $2/3 \times 1/20 \times 1/4$, which equals 1/120.

Sticklers for detail may argue that the derivation of the probability that II3 is a carrier has involved two minor errors. First, $2pq$ equals $2 \times 39/40 \times 1/40 = 0.04875 = 1/20.51$ rather than the value of 1/20 that was used. Second, the probability that an unaffected individual is a carrier equals $2pq/(p^2 + 2pq)$ $(= 0.04878)$ rather than $2pq/(p^2 + 2pq + q^2)$, since it is known that this individual is not affected.

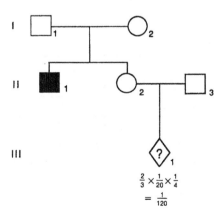

Figure 3.2. Risk to the healthy sibling of someone with cystic fibrosis for having an affected child (carrier frequency of cystic fibrosis is assumed to be 1 in 20).

Key Point 3

The probability that any two unaffected individuals will have a child with an autosomal recessive disorder equals the product of the probabilities that each is a carrier multiplied by 1/4.

For practical purposes, simply doubling the square root of the disease incidence is perfectly acceptable.

3.3 Risks to the Extended Family

Usually these risks will be very small. In Figure 3.3 values are given for the likelihood that various members of the extended family will be carriers. It is assumed that the parents of someone with an autosomal recessive disorder must be carriers; hence, their probability of heterozygosity is assigned as 1.0. Alternative possibilities such as uniparental disomy (p. 198) and new mutations are very unlikely and are therefore usually ignored. The likelihood of heterozygosity for other family members is halved for each degree of relationship removed from the parents. Strictly speaking, these probability values should be increased to take into account the additional possibility of heterozygosity due to inheritance of a different mutant allele from another ancestor, but usually this additional risk will be very small when compared with the much greater risk resulting from the genetic relationship to the affected homozygote. Consequently, this additional risk is usually ignored unless the carrier frequency of the disease in question is relatively high (see Section 3.7).

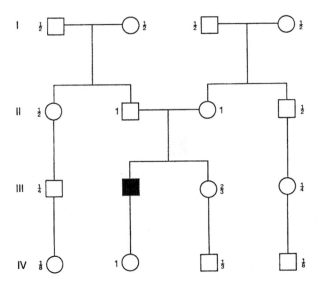

Figure 3.3. The probability of heterozygosity in relatives of someone with an autosomal recessive disorder.

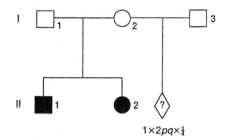

Figure 3.4. Risk to the half-sibling of someone with an autosomal recessive disorder. $2pq$ is the carrier frequency in the general population.

Key Point 4

The probability that a member of the extended pedigree is a carrier of an autosomal recessive disorder is halved for each degree of relationship removed from the parents.

Example 2

The parents of a child with an autosomal recessive disorder separate and wish to know the risk that each will have an affected child with a different partner. This can be calculated as $1 \times 2pq \times 1/4$, where $2pq$ equals the carrier frequency in the general population. This assumes that the new partner is healthy, unrelated, and with no family history of the relevant disorder. So for cystic fibrosis, assuming a carrier frequency of 1 in 20, the probability that the first child of individuals I2 and I3 in Figure 3.4 will be affected equals 1 in 80.

Example 3

This situation is similar to that discussed in Example 2, but now the couple seeking information (I2 and I3) already have two healthy children. Intuitively it can be seen that this makes it less likely that I3 is a carrier. This conditional information is taken into account using a Bayesian calculation (Table 3.4), from which it can be

Table 3.4. Risks to the Extended Family

Probability	Both I2 and I3 Are Carriers	I3 Is Not a Carrier
Prior	$\dfrac{1}{20}$	$\dfrac{19}{20}$
Conditional 2 healthy children	$\left(\dfrac{3}{4}\right)^2 = \dfrac{9}{16}$	1
Joint	$\dfrac{9}{320}$	$\dfrac{18}{20}$

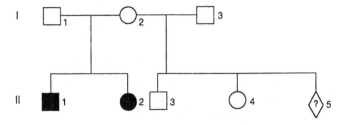

Figure 3.5. This relates to the same situation as in Figure 3.4, but the at-risk half-sibling already has two healthy full siblings.

shown that the posterior probability that both I2 and I3 are carriers (i.e., that I3 is a carrier) equals

$$\frac{9/320}{9/320 + 19/20}.$$

This approximates to 1/35, so the probability that the next child born to I2 and I3 in Figure 3.5 will be affected will be approximately $1/35 \times 1/4$, which equals 1/140. Clearly, this is substantially less than the 1/80 risk derived in Example 2.

Example 4

The sibling of someone with an autosomal recessive disorder marries a first cousin and wishes to know the probability that their first child will be affected. As indicated

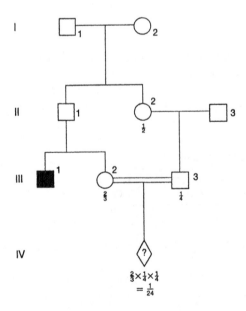

Figure 3.6. Risk to the offspring of a sibling of someone with an autosomal recessive disorder who marries a first cousin.

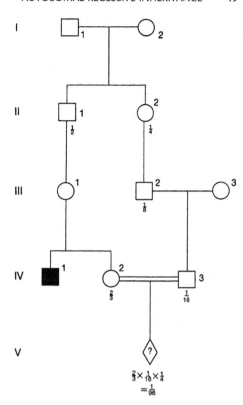

Figure 3.7. Risk to the offspring of a sibling of someone with an autosomal recessive disorder who marries a second cousin.

in Figure 3.6, this can be calculated relatively simply as $2/3 \times 1/4 \times 1/4$, which equals $1/24$.

Example 5

The sibling of someone with an autosomal recessive disorder marries a second cousin and wishes to know the probability that their first child will be affected. As shown in Figure 3.7, this can be calculated as $2/3 \times 1/16 \times 1/4$, which equals $1/96$.

3.4 Risks to the Offspring of an Affected Homozygote

Many individuals with autosomal recessive disorders marry and wish to have children. The child of any such union will be an obligatory heterozygote since he or she must inherit a mutant allele from the affected parent. Thus, the chance that a first child will be affected hinges on the probability that the unaffected parent is a carrier. The overall risk equals half of the probability of heterozygosity in the unaffected parent.

> **Key Point 5**
>
> The probability that a child born to an affected parent will also be affected equals half of the probability that the unaffected parent is a carrier.

Example 6

An individual with an autosomal recessive disorder has a healthy unrelated partner with no family history of the relevant condition. As shown in Figure 3.8, the probability that their first child will be affected will equal $1/2 \times 2pq = pq = q$ (as p approximates to 1), where $2pq$ equals the carrier frequency in the general population. Alternatively, the risk can be viewed as equal to the probability that the unaffected parent will transmit a mutant allele, which equals the gene frequency for mutant alleles in the population, i.e., q.

Example 7

An individual with a rare autosomal recessive disorder marries an unaffected first cousin. As shown in Figure 3.9, the probability of heterozygosity in the first cousin equals 1 in 4. Thus, the probability that the first child of this union will be affected equals $1/2 \times 1/4$, i.e., 1 in 8.

3.5 Two Brothers Marry Two Sisters

It is not uncommon in genetic counseling to encounter a large kindred in which two or more members of one sibship marry siblings from another unrelated sibship.

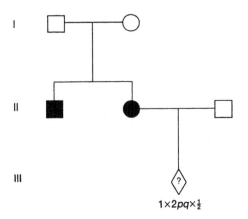

$1 \times 2pq \times \frac{1}{2}$

Figure 3.8. Risk to the offspring of a patient with an autosomal recessive disorder who marries a healthy unrelated individual. $2pq$ is the carrier frequency in the general population.

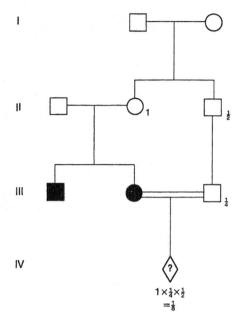

Figure 3.9. Risk to the offspring of a patient with an autosomal recessive disorder who marries a healthy first cousin.

$1 \times \frac{1}{4} \times \frac{1}{2}$
$= \frac{1}{8}$

Example 8

In this pedigree two sib pairs have married. One of these unions results in the birth of children with an autosomal recessive disorder. The other couple wish to know the probability that they will have an affected child. As shown in Figure 3.10, this can be calculated relatively simply as $1/2 \times 1/2 \times 1/4$, which equals 1 in 16.

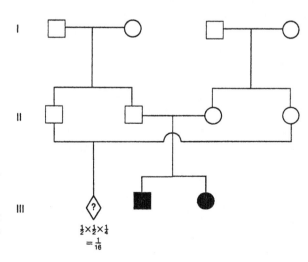

Figure 3.10. Two brothers have married two sisters. One marriage produces children with an autosomal recessive disorder. The risk to the first child of the other marriage is illustrated.

$\frac{1}{2} \times \frac{1}{2} \times \frac{1}{4}$
$= \frac{1}{16}$

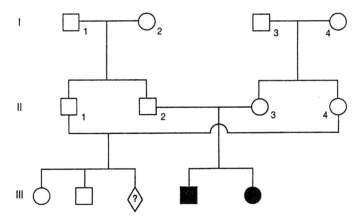

Figure 3.11. This relates to the same situation as in Figure 3.10, but the at-risk couple already have two healthy children.

Example 9

The pedigree in Figure 3.11 is essentially the same as that shown in Figure 3.10. However, the couple seeking information (II1 and II4) have already had two healthy children and wish to know the probability that a third child will be affected. This is calculated using Bayes' theorem to take into account the fact that the two normal offspring make it less likely that both II1 and II4 are carriers. The calculation is laid out as in Table 3.5. Here it can be seen that the posterior probability that both II1 and II4 are carriers equals $9/64/(9/64 + 48/64)$, which equals $9/57$. Therefore, the probability that their next child will be affected equals $9/57 \times 1/4$, which approximates to 1 in 25, a considerable decrease from the value of 1 in 16 that applied before the two unaffected children were born.

Table 3.5.

Probability	Both Parents Are (II1 and II4) Carriers	Only 1 Parent (II1 or II4) Is a Carrier or Both Are Not Carriers
Prior	$\dfrac{1}{4}$	$\dfrac{3}{4}$
Conditional 2 normal children	$\left(\dfrac{3}{4}\right)^2 = \dfrac{9}{16}$	1
Joint	$\dfrac{9}{64}$	$\dfrac{48}{64}$

Table 3.6.

Disease A	Disease B	Probability
Affected	Affected	$\frac{1}{4} \times \frac{1}{4} = \frac{1}{16}$
Affected	Not affected	$\frac{1}{4} \times \frac{3}{4} = \frac{3}{16}$
Not affected	Affected	$\frac{3}{4} \times \frac{1}{4} = \frac{3}{16}$
Not affected	Not affected	$\frac{3}{4} \times \frac{3}{4} = \frac{9}{16}$

3.6 Siblings with Different Autosomal Recessive Disorders

Example 10

If parents have had two children, each with a different autosomal recessive disorder, they may well wish to know the probability that a third child might inherit both, one, or neither of these conditions. To make the calculations manageable, it is assumed that the loci of the two disorders are not linked.

The calculation can be approached in a number of ways. First, we can consider in Table 3.6 the probabilities for the four possibilities for II3 in Figure 3.12. The same result can be achieved by simply calculating the probabilities that II3 would inherit both disorders ($1/4 \times 1/4$) or neither disorder ($3/4 \times 3/4$). This leaves a probability of $1 - (1/16 + 9/16) = 6/16$ that II3 will inherit only one disorder, i.e., $3/16$ for A but not B and $3/16$ for B but not A.

Alternatively, the solution can be arrived at more formally by using the binomial distribution (p. 8), using values of $p = 3/4$ and $q = 1/4$, where p and q equal the probabilities of not being affected and being affected, respectively.

If II3 in Figure 3.12 is not affected with either disorder, he or she may well wish to know the probability of heterozygosity for diseases A and/or B. These can be calculated relatively simply, as shown in Table 3.7. Thus, there is a probability of $8/9$ that the healthy sibling of II1 and II2 in Figure 3.12 will be a carrier of at least one of the two conditions.

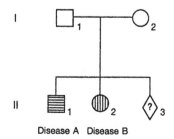

Figure 3.12. Healthy parents have two children, each with a different autosomal recessive disorder. The calculation that their next child will have either or both of these disorders is given in the text.

Table 3.7.

Disease A	Disease B	Probability
Heterozygous	Heterozygous	$\frac{2}{3} \times \frac{2}{3} = \frac{4}{9}$
Heterozygous	Homozygous unaffected	$\frac{2}{3} \times \frac{1}{3} = \frac{2}{9}$
Homozygous unaffected	Heterozygous	$\frac{1}{3} \times \frac{2}{3} = \frac{2}{9}$
Homozygous unaffected	Homozygous unaffected	$\frac{1}{3} \times \frac{1}{3} = \frac{1}{9}$

3.7 Allowing for Separate Mutations

In many of the situations considered so far (e.g., Examples 4 and 5), it has been assumed that the disorder is so rare that the likelihood of heterozygosity in family members due to inheritance of a different mutation is so low that it can be ignored. For most autosomal recessive disorders this is a reasonable assumption. However, if the disorder in question is relatively common, as is the case for cystic fibrosis, then an attempt should be made to allow for the possibility that a separate mutation is segregating independently in the family.

It is at this point that risk calculation for autosomal recessive disorders ceases to be straightforward. In the first edition of this book, a method was proposed for allowing for independent mutations by determining the possible genotypes for a particular relative in the following way. Consider the cousin (III 3) in Figure 3.6. There is 1 chance in 4 that this first cousin of an affected homozygote will be heterozygous for one of his affected cousin's mutations. This leaves a probability of 3 out of 4 that the gene inherited from their common grandparents will not be one of the affected cousin's mutant alleles. This enables the probabilities that the allele transmitted by II2 will be normal or mutant to be assigned as $\frac{3}{4}p$ and $\frac{3}{4}q$, respectively. Using this approach, it is possible to draw up a relatively simple table showing the possible different genotypes for the first cousin (Table 3.8). The overall probability that the cousin (III3) is a carrier equals the sum of the probability values for columns 2, 3, and 4 divided by the sum of probabilities 1 to 4 inclusive (columns 5 and 6 can be ignored, as it is known that III3 is not affected. This gives an overall probability of heterozygosity for III3 of

$$\frac{\frac{3}{4}pq + \frac{1}{4}p + \frac{3}{4}pq}{\frac{3}{4}p^2 + \frac{3}{4}pq + \frac{1}{4}p + \frac{3}{4}pq}$$

which reduces to

$$\frac{1 + 6q}{4 + 3q} \quad \text{as} \quad p = 1 - q$$

Table 3.8. Possible Genotypes for Individual III3 in Figure 3.6

	1	2	3	4	5	6
Maternally derived gene	Normal	Normal	Abnormal (same allele as III1)	Abnormal (different allele from III1)	Abnormal (same allele as III1)	Abnormal (different allele from III1)
	$\frac{3}{4}p$	$\frac{3}{4}p$	$\frac{1}{4}$	$\frac{3}{4}q$	$\frac{1}{4}$	$\frac{3}{4}q$
Paternally derived gene	Normal	Abnormal	Normal	Normal	Abnormal	Abnormal
	p	q	p	p	q	q
Genotype in III3	Homozygous normal	Heterozygous	Heterozygous	Heterozygous	Homozygous affected	Homozygous affected
Probability	$\frac{3}{4}p^2$	$\frac{3}{4}pq$	$\frac{1}{4}p$	$\frac{3}{4}pq$	$\frac{1}{4}q$	$\frac{3}{4}q^2$

Probability values are indicated for each event. For example, the probability that the maternally derived gene will be the same abnormal allele present in III1 equals 1/4; the probability that it will not be this allele equals 3/4.

Therefore, if $q = 1/40$ (assuming the incidence of cystic fibrosis, q^2, to be 1 in 1600), the probability that III3 is heterozygous can be calculated as 46/163 or 0.282, instead of the figure of 0.25, which is obtained by ignoring the possibility of separate mutations. For values of $q = 1/100$ (e.g., phenylketonuria) and 1/500 (e.g., ataxia-telangiectasia), the probability that III3 is heterozygous equals 0.263 and 0.253, respectively.

If this method is used to calculate the carrier risk for a second cousin, then a value of $(1 + 30q)/(16 + 15q)$ is obtained. For values of $q = 1/40$, 1/100, and 1/500 this gives carrier risks of 0.107, 0.08, and 0.066, respectively compared with the figure of $0.0625 (= 1/16)$, which is obtained if separate mutations are ignored.

The advantage of this approach is that it is relatively straightforward. The problem is that it does not take into account pedigree information that "tests" whether other mutations could be present. For example, in Figure 3.6 the fact that I1, I2, II1, and II2 are unaffected should be taken into consideration. Similarly, if I1 and I2 had other unaffected children, then this information should also be incorporated into the calculation.

This means that ideally a Bayesian calculation should be undertaken for each individual family. Realistically, this is impractical, particularly if the results of selective mutation testing are to be incorporated, unless a specifically designed computer program is readily available (Curnow, 1994). An illustration of how each calculation should be undertaken is given in the following example.

Example 11

The problem is to calculate the risk that the first cousin (III3) in Figure 3.6 is a carrier, taking into account the possibility of separate mutations and all pedigree information. The first step is to construct a Bayesian table to determine the carrier

Table 3.9. (see Fig. 3.6 and Example 11).

Probability	I1 and I2 Are Both Carriers		Either I1 or I2 Is a Carrier But Not Both	
Prior	$2pq \times 2pq = 4p^2q^2$		$2 \times p^2 \times 2pq = 4p^3q$	
Conditional				
III1 is a carrier	$\dfrac{1}{2}$		$\dfrac{1}{2}$	
II2 is not affected	C	NC	C	NC
	$\dfrac{1}{2}$	$\dfrac{1}{4}$	$\dfrac{1}{2}$	$\dfrac{1}{2}$
Joint	p^2q^2	$\dfrac{1}{2}p^2q^2$	p^3q	p^3q

Posterior probability that II2 is a carrier $= (p^2q^2 + p^3q)/\left(p^2q^2 + \dfrac{1}{2}p^2q^2 + p^3q + p^3q\right)$ (1)

$$= (q + p)/\left(q + \dfrac{1}{2}q + 2p\right) \quad \text{(divide (1) by } p^2q)$$

$$= 1/((2 - q)/2) \quad \text{(as } p + q = 1)$$

Table 3.10. (see Fig. 3.6 and Example 11).

Probability	Both II2 and II3 Are Carriers		II2 Is a Carrier II3 Is Not a Carrier		II3 Is a Carrier II2 Is Not a Carrier		Both II2 and II3 Are Not Carriers	
Prior	$C_M 2pq$		$C_M p^2$		$2pq(1 - C_M)$		$(1 - C_M)p^2$	
Conditional								
III1	C	NC	C	NC	C	NC	C	NC
(III1 is not affected)	$\frac{1}{2}$	$\frac{1}{4}$	$\frac{1}{2}$	$\frac{1}{2}$	$\frac{1}{2}$	$\frac{1}{2}$	0	1
Joint	a	b	c	d	e	f	g	h

Posterior probability that III1 is a carrier $= (a + c + e + g)/(a + b + c + d + e + f + g + h)$

$$= (C_M + 2Q - C_M q)/(2 + 2q - C_M q)$$

risk for II2, the mother of III3 (Table 3.9). By simple algebra this can be shown to reduce to $1/(2 - q/2)$.

The next step is to determine the probability that III3 is a carrier given that the probability that his mother is a carrier equals $1/(2 - q/2)$, which we shall notate as C_M, and that the probability that his father is a carrier equals $2pq$, this being the carrier frequency in the general population. To achieve this, another Bayesian table is drawn up (Table 3.10). From this it can be shown that the probability that III3 is heterozygous equals

$$\frac{C_M + 2q - C_M q}{2 + 2q - C_M q}$$

This yields carrier risks of 0.265, 0.256, and 0.251 for values of $q = 1/40$, $1/100$, and $1/500$, respectively. As expected, these values are slightly lower than the values of 0.282, 0.263, and 0.253 obtained using the previous method. In the same way, it can be shown that the probability that a second cousin, such as IV3 in Figure 3.7, is a carrier equals 0.095, 0.0765, and 0.065 for values of $q =$

Key Point 6

When calculating the risk that the relative of an affected homozygote is a carrier, some consideration should be given to the possibility that other mutant alleles are present in the family. This is not important when the gene frequency is low. When the gene frequency is high, this makes only a small difference to the probability of heterozygosity for close relatives (e.g., 0.265 instead of 0.25 for a first cousin). For more distant relatives, the more remote relationship permits a much greater chance of heterozygosity due to inheritance of a separate mutation (e.g., 0.095 instead of 0.0625 for a second cousin). For very distant relatives, an approximation of the probability of heterozygosity can be obtained by adding the general population carrier frequency to the probability resulting from the relationship with the affected proband.

1/40, 1/100, and 1/500, respectively. Once again these are slightly lower than the values of 0.107, 0.08, and 0.066 obtained previously.

3.8 Consanguinity

Several pedigrees featuring consanguinity with a known autosomal recessive disorder in the family have already been considered, e.g., Figures 3.6, 3.7, and 3.9. In these examples the probability of homozygosity in a child was calculated by establishing the nature of the mating (i.e., affected versus possible carrier or possible carrier versus possible carrier) and the probability of heterozygosity in the possible carriers.

A similar approach is employed when assessing risks to the offspring of consanguineous couples with no history of autosomal recessive disease in the family. Toward this end, it is usually assumed that everyone carries one gene for a serious autosomal recessive handicapping disorder, an assumption based on the study of the offspring of consanguineous marriages (Bittles and Neel, 1994; Jaber et al., 1998). It may well be that the average human also carries several lethal recessive genes resulting in early pregnancy loss, but the point can reasonably be made that individuals seeking genetic counseling are much more concerned about possible long-term handicapping disorders in a surviving child than the possible risk of first trimester miscarriage. Therefore, the probability that the first child of a consanguineous marriage will have a serious autosomal recessive disorder due to homozygosity by descent from a common ancestor is usually calculated on the assumption that each common ancestor of the consanguineous couple seeking information carried one deleterious autosomal recessive gene.

Coefficient of Inbreeding

At this stage, it is appropriate to introduce some potentially confusing definitions. Frequent mention is made of the *coefficient of inbreeding* (F) in textbooks of population genetics. This is defined as the probability that the child of a consanguineous marriage will be homozygous for a specific gene derived from a common ancestor. Such alleles are described as being "identical by descent," and the homozygous state is referred to as "autozygous." Values for F for the children of various relationships are given in Table 3.11. This table also includes values for the

---

Key Point 7

The coefficient of inbreeding (F) relates to the *child* of a consanguineous relationship and indicates the probability that the child will be homozygous for a specific gene derived from a common ancestor. The coefficient of relationship (R) relates to a consanguineous *couple* and indicates the proportion of genes that on average they would be expected to share by descent from common ancestors.

Table 3.11. Coefficients of Relationship and Inbreeding Plus Risk to Offspring for Autosomal Recessive Disease.

Relationship	Coefficient of Relationship R	Coefficient of Inbreeding F	Risk of Autosomal Recessive Disease in Offspring*
Siblings	$\frac{1}{2}$	$\frac{1}{4}$	$\frac{1}{8}$
Half siblings	$\frac{1}{4}$	$\frac{1}{8}$	$\frac{1}{16}$
Uncle–niece, aunt–nephew	$\frac{1}{4}$	$\frac{1}{8}$	$\frac{1}{16}$
First cousins	$\frac{1}{8}$	$\frac{1}{16}$	$\frac{1}{32}$
First cousins once removed	$\frac{1}{16}$	$\frac{1}{32}$	$\frac{1}{64}$
Second cousins	$\frac{1}{32}$	$\frac{1}{64}$	$\frac{1}{128}$
Double first cousins	$\frac{1}{4}$	$\frac{1}{8}$	$\frac{1}{16}$
Double second cousins	$\frac{1}{16}$	$\frac{1}{32}$	$\frac{1}{64}$

*Assuming each common ancestor carried one deleterious autosomal recessive gene.

coefficient of relationship (R), which indicates the proportion of genes shared by individuals who are relatives.

The coefficient of inbreeding (F) for the child of first cousins is stated as being 1/16, which by definition is the probability of homozygosity for a specific allele derived from a common ancestor in the child of first cousins. The value of 1/16 is derived by calculating the probability that the child of a first cousin marriage will be homozygous for either allele 1 or 2 in the common parental grandfather or allele 1 or 2 in the common parental grandmother. The value for each of these probabilities is 1 in 64. Thus, the value for F of 1/16 is obtained by summing the value for each locus specific allele. Alternatively, the value of 1/16 can be derived by considering that if one parent in a first-cousin marriage transmits a particular gene to a child, then the probability that the other parent will transmit the same gene equals $R \times 1/2 = 1/8 \times 1/2 = 1/16$.

For counseling purposes this is potentially misleading, since we are interested only in the probability of homozygosity for each parent's bad allele, not the good allele also. Thus, the value of interest to the first-cousin parents will be 1/32, which equals F multiplied by 1/2 (i.e., divided by 2). Hence, as a generalization, it can be concluded that the probability that the child of a consanguineous mating will have a serious autosomal recessive disorder as a consequence of homozygosity due to descent from a common ancestor equals $F/2$. If in the future, if it is discovered that each human carries more than one severe autosomal recessive gene, say n, then the risk to the offspring of a consanguineous union will be $(F/2) \times n$.

Key Point 8

The probability that a child born to consanguineous parents will have an autosomal recessive disorder equals $(F/2) \times n$, where n equals the average number of recessive alleles carried by each common ancestor.

Example 12

First cousins with no family history of autosomal recessive disease wish to know the probability that their first child will have a serious autosomal recessive disorder as a consequence of their genetic relationship. It is assumed that each of their common grandparents (I1 and I2) carried one deleterious gene. Thus, the probability that both III1 and III2 carry their common grandfather's deleterious gene equals $1/4 \times 1/4$, so the probability of homozygosity for this gene in their first child will be $1/4 \times 1/4 \times 1/4$, which equals $1/64$. A similar exercise is undertaken for the common grandmother, I2. Thus, the total probability of homozygosity for a deleterious autosomal recessive disorder in the first child of III1 and III2 in Figure 3.13 will be $1/64 + 1/64$, which equals $1/32$.

Example 13

Awareness of potential risks associated with marriage within the family prompts many consanguineous couples to seek information about the likelihood that they

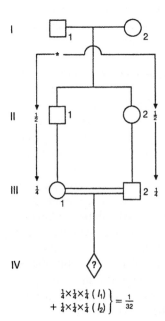

$$\left.\begin{array}{l} \tfrac{1}{4} \times \tfrac{1}{4} \times \tfrac{1}{4} \, (I_1) \\ + \tfrac{1}{4} \times \tfrac{1}{4} \times \tfrac{1}{4} \, (I_2) \end{array}\right\} = \tfrac{1}{32}$$

Figure 3.13. The probability that the first child of first cousins will have an autosomal recessive disorder as a consequence of homozygosity by descent from a common ancestor.

might have a child with a disorder that shows a high incidence in their particular population. In this example, prospective parents who are first cousins wish to know the probability that their first child will be affected with cystic fibrosis. The carrier frequency in their population is 1 in 20, and neither of the cousins has a family history of cystic fibrosis.

One approach to this question is to draw up a Bayesian table to take into account all relevant family members who could influence the probability that one or both of the first cousins could be carriers. As indicated in Example 11, this can be extremely difficult and certainly cannot be carried out quickly on the back of the proverbial envelope at a busy peripheral clinic. As a compromise, it is possible to use a little simple algebra based on the assumption that the risk will equal the sum of the general population incidence (q^2) plus the risk resulting from the consanguinity. In the case of first cousins, this equals the probability that one of the two common grandparents is a carrier (i.e., $2 \times 2pq$) multiplied by the probability that a child of first cousins will be homozygous by descent from one grandparent, i.e., 1 in 64 (Fig. 3.13). This gives an overall risk of $q^2 + (4pq \times 1/64) = q^2 + (pq \times 1/16)$. Note that this can also be expressed as $q^2 + Fpq$, as F for first cousins equals 1/16. For a value of $q = 1/40$, as in cystic fibrosis, this gives an overall risk of approximately 1 in 465. For second cousins ($F = 1/64$), the risk that a child will have cystic fibrosis equals $q^2 + Fpq =$ approximately 1 in 994.

These risks will be substantially reduced if molecular testing fails to identify a common mutation in either of the cousin partners. This is considered further in the next section (Example 18).

Example 14

Knowledge of the value of the coefficient of inbreeding is further illustrated by the potentially confusing situation illustrated in Figure 3.14. In this pedigree, III1 and

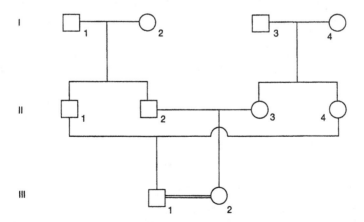

Figure 3.14. Individuals III1 and III2 are first cousins through their fathers and through their mothers. Hence they are double first cousins.

III2 are first cousins through their fathers, who are siblings. They are also first cousins through their mothers, who are also siblings. Therefore, III1 and III2 are double first cousins.

Assuming that each common ancestor carried one deleterious autosomal recessive mutation, the probability that the first child of III1 and III2 will be autozygous and therefore affected equals 1/64 for each of these common ancestors, giving a total of 1/16. This figure can be obtained very quickly by simply halving the value of F (1/8) given in Table 3.11.

Example 15

In the pedigree shown in Figure 3.15, IV1 and IV2 are double second cousins. The probability that their first child will be autozygous for the deleterious gene of each common great-great-grandparent (generation I) will be $1/8 \times 1/8 \times 1/4$, which equals 1/256, giving a total probability of 1/64. The same value can be obtained by halving the F value of 1/32 given in Table 3.11.

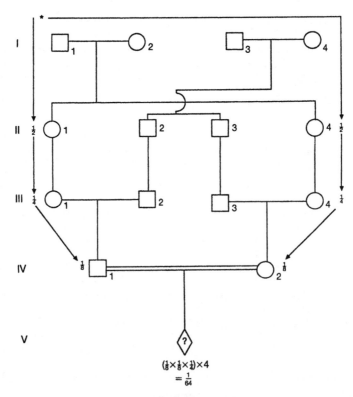

Figure 3.15. In this pedigree, individuals IV1 and IV2 are double second cousins. The probability that their first child will be homozygous by descent from a common great-great-grandparent in generation I will be 1/256. Since there are four common great-great-grandparents, the total probability of homozygosity equals $1/256 \times 1/4 = 1/64$.

Example 16

Examples 14 and 15 illustrate the basic approach to determining risks in consanguineous pedigrees. Essentially this involves identifying all common ancestors and then calculating the probability of autozygosity in the at-risk individual for each of these ancestors. Thus, in Example 14, there were four common ancestors (I1, I2, I3, and I4), with the probability of autozygosity for each equaling 1 in 64, giving a total of 1 in 16. As an alternative, an assessment of risk can be made using the coefficient of inbreeding, F, by identifying independent relationships in the parents of the at-risk child that could lead to autozygosity. In Example 14 these consisted of two sets of first cousins.

In more complex pedigrees it can be very difficult to use this latter approach, so it is usually necessary to identify all relevant founder common ancestors and then establish the different pathways down the pedigree through which the child of the concerned prospective parents could be autozygous. A *founder* common ancestor is one whose parents are not in the pedigree and who could transmit his or her deleterious gene to each of the prospective parents.

Figure 3.16 shows an example of the type of complex pedigree that can be encountered in a large inbred kindred. To enhance understanding, the family members have all been given names. The presenting couple, Deb and Don, wish to know the probability that their first child will have an autosomal recessive disorder as a consequence of the strong family history of consanguinity. This is determined by drawing up a table of all the possible ways in which their child

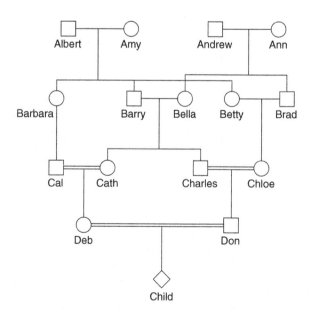

Figure 3.16. A family pedigree showing complex consanguinity. What is the probability that the child born to Deb and Don will have an autosomal recessive disorder?

Table 3.12. (see Fig. 3.16 and Example 16)

Common Founder Ancestor	Pathways	Probability
Albert	1. Barbara–Cal–Deb–Child Barry–Charles–Don–Child	$\left(\dfrac{1}{2}\right)^8$
	2. Barbara–Cal–Deb–Child Betty–Chloe–Don–Child	$\left(\dfrac{1}{2}\right)^8$
	3. Barry–Cath–Deb–Child Betty–Chloe–Don–Child	$\left(\dfrac{1}{2}\right)^8$
	4. Barry–Cath–Deb–Child –Charles–Don–Child	$\left(\dfrac{1}{2}\right)^7$
Amy	As for Albert, i.e.,	$\left(3 \times \left(\dfrac{1}{2}\right)^8\right) + \left(\dfrac{1}{2}\right)^7$
Andrew	1. Bella–Cath–Deb–Child Brad–Chloe–Don–Child	$\left(\dfrac{1}{2}\right)^8$
	2. Bella–Cath–Deb–Child –Charles–Don–Child	$\left(\dfrac{1}{2}\right)^7$
Ann	As for Andrew, i.e.,	$\left(\dfrac{1}{2}\right)^8 + \left(\dfrac{1}{2}\right)^7$

The total probability that the child will be autozygous $= (8 \times (1/2)^8) + (4 \times (1/2)^7) = (1/2)^4 = 1$ in 16.

could be autozygous (Table 3.12). The overall risk for their first child can be calculated to be 1 in 16, assuming that each of the four founder common ancestors carried a single deleterious autosomal recessive allele. This is consistent with the coefficient of inbreeding for this child equaling 1/8, indicating that the genetic relationship between Deb and Don is identical to that between an uncle and niece (Table 3.11).

3.9 Direct Mutation Analysis and Multiple Alleles

In the examples considered so far, it has been assumed that there are only two alleles—wild type and mutant—at each locus. For many disorders multiple alleles exist, the best-known example being cystic fibrosis, for which over 1000 different mutations have been identified. A screening test for the most common mutations detects approximately 90% of all carriers with the most common mutation, known as ΔF508, accounting for around 75% of all cystic fibrosis alleles in Western Europe

Table 3.13. (see Example 17).

Probability	Carrier	Not a Carrier
Prior	1/20	19/20
Conditional		
Negative screening test	1/10	1
Joint	1/200	19/20

Posterior carrier probability $= 1/200/(1/200 + 19/20) = 1/191$

(Ferrie et al., 1992). Applying this technology in practice can generate some very difficult calculations.

Example 17

What is the probability that a healthy member of the general population is a carrier of cystic fibrosis if he/she tests negative on the common mutation screening analysis? The incidence of cystic fibrosis in the general population is 1 in 1600, and the common mutation screening test detects 90% of all cystic fibrosis alleles.

The answer is obtained by drawing up a simple Bayesian table (Table 3.13). The posterior probability that a healthy member of the general population is a carrier, given a negative common mutation screening test, is $1/200$ divided by $1/200 + 19/20$, which equals 1 in 191. Table 3.14 shows the same calculation, but instead the carrier frequency in the general population is denoted as x and the proportion of carriers who test positive on the common mutation screening test is denoted as y. The posterior probability that an individual who tests negative is a carrier equals $(x - xy)/(1 - xy)$.

Example 18

In Example 13, we considered the risk that a consanguineous couple might have a child with a specific autosomal recessive disorder and showed that this can

Table 3.14. (see Example 17).

Probability	Carrier	Not a Carrier
Prior	x	$1-x$
Conditional		
Negative mutation screen	$1-y$	1
Joint	$x(1-y)$	$1-x$

Posterior probability that individual is a carrier given negative mutation screen $=$
$x(1 - y)/(x(1 - y) + 1 - x) = (x - xy)/(1 - xy)$

> **Key Point 9**
>
> By substituting x for the carrier frequency in the general population and y for the proportion of carriers who test positive on screening in Table 3.13, it can be shown that the probability that an individual who tests negative is a carrier equals $(x - xy)/(1 - xy)$. This general formula can be used for any situation in which a prior probability (x) of an event, such as carrier frequency or gene frequency, is reduced by a screening test result that identifies a proportion (y) of the relevant carriers or mutations.

be calculated for any relationship as $q^2 + Fpq$, where q equals the frequency of the mutant allele, p equals the frequency of the normal (wild-type allele), and F equals the coefficient of inbreeding for the parents. In this example, first-cousin parents are concerned about the risk that they might have a child with cystic fibrosis, and their carrier risk has been modified by the common mutation screen for which they have both tested negative. What is the residual probability that they will have an affected child?

The probability that these parents will have an affected child is modified by substituting new values for p and q in the formula $q^2 + Fpq$. Using the formula given in Key Point 9, the gene frequency for nonidentifiable mutations falls from its prior value of 1/40 to 1/391. This means that the probability that their first child will be affected equals $(1/391)^2 + (1/16 \times 390/391 \times 1/391)$, which equals approximately 1 in 6025.

Example 19

A healthy woman (II2 in Fig. 3.17) wishes to know the probability that she and her healthy unrelated partner (II3) will have a child with spinal muscular atrophy. Her concern is based on the fact that she had an affected brother (II1) who died in childhood and who was shown to be homozygous for the common *SMN1* gene deletion. Both the woman and her partner undergo testing for this common deletion. The woman is found to be a carrier. Her partner tests negative. The incidence of spinal muscular atrophy in the general population is 1 in 10,000, and the common

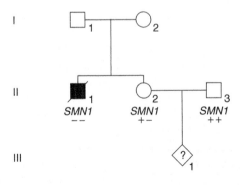

Figure 3.17. What is the probability that the first child born to II2 and II3 will be affected with spinal muscular atrophy? *SMN1* = survival motor neuron gene.

Table 3.15. (see Example 19).

Probability	II3 Is a Carrier	II3 Is Not a Carrier
Prior	$1/50 = 0.02$	$49/50 = 0.98$
Conditional		
Negative mutation screen	0.06	1
Joint	$\overline{0.0012}$	$\overline{0.98}$

Posterior probability that II3 is a carrier $= 0.0012/(0.0012 + 0.98) = 1$ in 818 (approximately)

deletion accounts for 94% of all mutations. What is the probability that her partner is a carrier, and what is the probability that their first child will be affected?

The answer is provided by constructing a Bayesian table (Table 3.15), which indicates that the posterior probability that the partner is a carrier equals approximately 1 in 818. The same answer can be obtained by substituting 0.02 for x and 0.94 for y in the formula $(x - xy)/(1 - xy)$. This means that the probability that the first child born to this woman and her partner will be affected equals 1 (the carrier probability for II2) $\times$ 1/818 (the carrier probability for II3) $\times$ 1/4 (the probability that a child born to two carriers will be affected), giving an overall risk of 1 in 3272. More complex examples of determining carrier risks and mutation testing in spinal muscular atrophy are provided by Ogino et al. (2002).

3.10 Case Scenario

Figure 3.18 shows a simple pedigree in which the sister of a boy who has died with a clinically confirmed diagnosis of cystic fibrosis wishes to know the probability that she and her healthy unrelated partner will have an affected child. Unfortunately, no DNA is available from either the deceased boy or his father. Using the common mutation screening test, it emerges that the mother, I2, is a carrier of the common ΔF508 deletion mutation. The sister, II2, tests negative on the common mutation

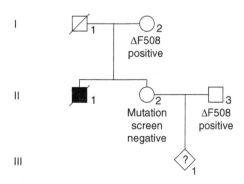

Figure 3.18. What is the probability that the first child born to II2 and II3 will be affected with cystic fibrosis?

Table 3.16. (see case scenario).

Probability	Father Detectable Mutation	Mother ΔFpos	Father Undetectable Mutation	Mother ΔFpos
Prior	9		1	
Conditional				
II2	C	NC	C	NC
Prior	1/2	1/4	1/2	1/4
Conditional				
Mutation	0	1	1/2	1
screen negative				
Joint	0	9/4	1/4	1/4

Posterior probability that II2 is a carrier $= 1/4/(9/4 + 1/4 + 1/4) = 1/11$.

screen. Her partner is also found to be a carrier of the ΔF508 deletion. What is the probability that II2 is a carrier, given that the screening test identifies 90% of all mutations, and what is the probability that their first child will be affected?

To demonstrate the versatility of Bayesian analysis three different tables are shown, all of which indicate that the carrier risk for the sister, II2, has fallen from 2 in 3 to 1 in 11. Table 3.16 uses prior probabilities based on the combined possible parental genotypes; the prior probability that the father, I1, had a mutation that would be detectable on screening is nine times the probability that his mutation would be undetectable. Table 3.17 considers the prior probabilities based on the possible carrier status of II2. Table 3.18 is similar, but the conditional probabilities have been combined by adding the probabilities that the sister would test negative if she had inherited either her mother's mutation or her father's mutation. In practice, it does not matter which type of table is constructed as long as all prior probabilities are considered and all relevant information is used once and only once (p. 14).

Table 3.17. (see case scenario).

Probability	II2 Is a Carrier		II2 Is Not a Carrier
	Paternal Mutation	Maternal Mutation	
Prior	1/3	1/3	1/3
Conditional			
Negative mutation	1/10	0	1
screen			
Joint	1/30	0	1/3

Posterior probability that II2 is a carrier $= 1/30/(1/30 + 1/3) = 1/11$

Table 3.18. (see case scenario).

Probability	II2 Is a Carrier	II2 Is Not a Carrier
Prior	2/3	1/3
Conditional		
Mutation screen negative	$1/2(\text{mat}) \times 0$ $+ 1/2(\text{pat}) \times 1/10$ $= 1/20$	1
Joint	$\overline{1/30}$	$\overline{1/3}$

Posterior probability that II2 is a carrier $= 1/30/(1/30 + 1/3) = 1/11$

Based on this carrier risk for II2 of 1 in 11, she and her partner can be informed that the probability that their first child will be affected equals 1/11 (the carrier probability for II2) $\times$ 1 (the carrier probability for II3) $\times$ 1/4 (the probability that two carriers will have an affected child), which equals 1 in 44.

Further Reading

Bridge, P.J. (1997). *The calculation of genetic risks. Worked examples in DNA diagnostics* (2nd ed.). Johns Hopkins University Press, Baltimore and London.

Ogino, S., Wilson, R.B., Gold, B., Hawley, P., and Grody, W.W. (2004). Bayesian analysis for cystic fibrosis risks in prenatal and carrier screening. *Genetics in Medicine*, **6**, 439–449.

Spence, M.A. and Hodge, S.E. (2000). The "circular" problems of calculating risk: dealing with consanguinity. *Journal of Genetic Counseling*, **9**, 179–201.

4

X-Linked Recessive Inheritance

In X-linked recessive inheritance the condition is manifest in the male, who is described as being *hemizygous*, whereas, by definition, the heterozygous carrier female is not affected, although careful examination or appropriate investigations may occasionally reveal subtle abnormalities. When a female is known to be a carrier, then each of her sons has a 50% risk of inheriting the disorder in question, and each of her daughters has a 50% risk of being a carrier. When an affected male reproduces, all of his daughters will be carriers, as they will all have inherited his X chromosome, and all of his sons will be unaffected, as they must have inherited his Y chromosome.

Unfortunately, the calculation of risks for X-linked recessive disorders is rarely as easy as this simple outline suggests. For example, if an affected male represents an isolated case in a family, then it is essential to try to establish whether he represents a new mutation or whether his mother is a carrier. The existence of unaffected uncles, brothers, and nephews has to be taken into account, as do the results of appropriate carrier tests undertaken not only on the mother but also on other close female relatives in the matrilineal line.

Various methods have been devised to tackle the difficult calculations that can arise, and several excellent computer programs can be used to assist the reluctant mathematician (Flodman and Hodge, 2002). The examples that follow have been selected to illustrate how quite difficult pedigrees can be assessed without recourse to the microchip. For the sake of consistency and in keeping with the user-friendly ethos of this book, the general approach used throughout this chapter will be the same. This relies heavily on the construction of a Bayesian table that takes into account all possible genotypes and compares their joint probabilities to give a posterior or absolute probability for carrier status.

This approach has been used elsewhere in this book and has been described in general terms in Chapter 1. Readers who have difficulty coming to terms with

Bayesian tables may prefer to try alternative methods. These include the use of likelihood ratios (Jeanpierre, 1988), probability trees (Friedman and Fish, 1980) and probability products (Maag and Gold, 1975). Fundamentally these methods are very similar, differing principally in the way in which the data are set out.

In several of the following examples, a technique involving the use of a *dummy consultand* is employed. The dummy consultand is usually the nearest female ancestor common to both the affected male and the female seeking information, who is known as the *true consultand* or simply as the *consultand*. Often the dummy consultand will be the mother or grandmother of the true consultand. Thus, the principle employed is to calculate a provisional posterior probability for the dummy consultand and then use this to derive a prior probability for the true consultand.

In Examples 1–6 it is assumed that the mutation rates in male and female gametogenesis are equal. In Examples 1–10 risks are calculated on the basis that the biological fitness of affected males is zero, so that the possibility that an affected male will transmit a mutant gene to a daughter can be ignored.

4.1 The Prior Probability That a Female Is a Carrier of an X-Linked Recessive Disorder

Bayesian analysis is based on modification of prior probabilities, so that when estimating genetic risks for X-linked recessive disorders, it is necessary to assign a prior probability that a woman is a carrier of a particular disorder. Sometimes this will be based on the pedigree structure, but in many instances the prior probability will be that which applies to all women in the population. It is widely stated in textbooks that there is a prior probability of 4μ that any female is a carrier of a particular X-linked recessive disorder with genetic fitness of zero, but how this value has been derived is not always clear. The explanation favored by this author is as follows.

Figure 4.1 represents a pedigree showing direct female descendants of Adam and Eve (I1 and I2). The mutation rates in females and males are denoted as μ and v, respectively. It is assumed that Adam did not have the relevant disorder and that Eve did not carry it. Thus, the probability that their daughter in generation II will be a carrier equals $\mu + v$, i.e., the likelihood of an X chromosome mutation occurring in the female or male germ cell. The probability that the daughter in generation III will be a carrier equals half of her mother's probability plus μ plus v. Extending this process to generation N, it becomes apparent that there will be a prior probability of 2μ plus $2v$ that the female descendant in generation N is a carrier. If the mutation rate is the same in males and females, then this value will equal 4μ. Note that throughout this procedure the possibility that an affected male will transmit the abnormal gene can be ignored since biological (= genetic) fitness of males equals zero.

This value of 4μ can be derived more conventionally by considering that the incidence of carrier females in generation $n + 1$ (C_{n+1}) will equal half of the incidence of carrier females in the previous generation (C_n) plus the sum of the mutation rates in males (v) and females (μ), i.e., $C_{n+1} = 1/2\,C_n + \mu + v$.

At equilibrium $C_{n+1} = C_n$. Therefore, $C_{n+1} = 2\mu + 2v = 4\mu$ if $\mu = v$.

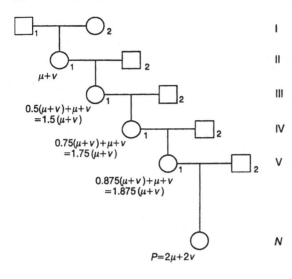

Figure 4.1. This shows the derivation of the probability (P) that any female is a carrier of a specific X-linked recessive disorder in which affected males have fitness = 0. μ and v are the mutation rates in female and male germ cells.

Key Point 1

There is a prior probability of 4μ that a female is a carrier of an X-linked recessive disorder for which affected males have a genetic fitness of zero and the mutation rates in males and females are equal.

4.2 The Probability That the Mother of an Isolated Case Is a Carrier

The information derived in Section 4.1 can be used to determine the probability that the mother or grandmother of an isolated case is a carrier. Figure 4.2 shows the simplest possible pedigree of a grandmother, mother, and affected son. The estimation of probabilities is achieved as shown in Table 4.1.

In this table it can be seen that the posterior probability that the grandmother I1 is a carrier equals $\frac{\mu + 2\mu^2}{\mu + 2\mu^2 + \mu + \mu}$, which reduces to 1/3 if $2\mu^2$ is ignored.

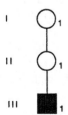

Figure 4.2. The provisional probability that the mother and grandmother are carriers equals 2/3 and 1/3, respectively. See the text for derivation of these values.

Table 4.1.

Probability	I1 Is a Carrier		I1 Is Not a Carrier	
Prior II1	4μ Carrier	Not carrier	$1-4\mu=1$ Carrier	Not carrier
Prior	$\dfrac{1}{2}$	$\dfrac{1}{2}$	2μ	1
Conditional 1 affected son	$\dfrac{1}{2}$	μ	$\dfrac{1}{2}$	μ
Joint	μ	$2\mu^2$	μ	μ

Similarly the posterior probability that the mother II1 is a carrier equals $\dfrac{\mu+\mu}{\mu+2\mu^2+\mu+\mu}$, which reduces to 2/3 if $2\mu^2$ is ignored.

(Note that in all calculations μ^2 or μ^3 will be ignored throughout this chapter since, as μ is a small number in the region of 1×10^{-5} or less, μ^2 or μ^3 will be negligible.)

These values of 2/3 and 1/3 can be used to shortcut some of the more laborious calculations that can arise as illustrated in Example 1, but generally shortcuts should be avoided since they increase the scope for error.

4.3 The Carrier Risks For Female Relatives of an Isolated Case

This is an issue that arises frequently in clinical practice. In the following examples, increasingly complex pedigrees will be considered to show how family structure in the matrilineal line should be taken into account.

Example 1: A Nuclear Family

In Figure 4.3, II1 represents an isolated case of an X-linked recessive disorder, and his sister, II2, wishes to know the likelihood that she is a carrier. If the mother, I2, is known to be a carrier, perhaps because she had an affected brother, then there would be a prior probability of 1 in 2 that II2 is a carrier. However, the fact that II1 is an isolated case means that the possibility that he represents a new mutation has to be taken into account. To achieve this, his mother's prior probability for being a carrier is assigned as 4μ and the calculation proceeds as in Table 4.2.

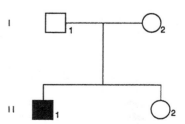

Figure 4.3. II2 is the consultand.

Table 4.2.

Probability	I2 Is a Carrier	I2 Is Not a Carrier
Prior	4μ	$1 - 4\mu = 1$
Conditional		
1 affected son	$\dfrac{1}{2}$	μ
Joint	2μ	μ

This indicates that the posterior probability that I2 is a carrier equals $2\mu/3\mu$, which equals 2/3 . The prior probability that the sister, II2, is a carrier equals half of her mother's posterior probability for being a carrier, i.e., 1/3.

Example 2: Incorporating Unaffected Brothers

Once again, the sister of an isolated case is the consultand, but in this example, (Fig. 4.4) she also has two unaffected brothers. The calculation proceeds as in Table 4.3. The posterior probability that I2 is a carrier equals $(\mu/2)/(\mu/2 + \mu)$, which equals 1/3 , so that the prior probability that II4 is a carrier equals 1/6.

The same answer could have been obtained by working on the basis that there is a prior probability of 2/3 that I2 is a carrier since she is the mother of an isolated case (Table 4.4). Thus, this also yields a posterior probability of 1/6 /(1/6 + 1/3), which equals 1/3 , that I2 is a carrier. Note that in this latter shortcut approach, no account is taken of the affected son under conditional probabilities since this information has already been used when assigning his mother's prior probability as 2/3. Once again, this illustrates one of the most important principles of Bayesian calculations, i.e., *information must never be used twice.*

Key Point 2

Information about the structure of the nuclear family can be incorporated in a Bayesian table in which each unaffected brother provides conditional probabilities of $\frac{1}{2}$ to 1 for the mother being a carrier versus not being a carrier.

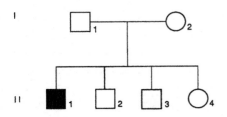

Figure 4.4. II4 is the consultand.

Table 4.3.

Probability	I2 Is a Carrier	I2 Is Not a Carrier
Prior	4μ	$1 - 4\mu = 1$
Conditional		
1 affected son	$\dfrac{1}{2}$	μ
2 unaffected sons	$\dfrac{1}{4}$	1
Joint	$\mu/2$	μ

Table 4.4.

Probability	I2 Is a Carrier	I2 Is Not a Carrier
Prior	$\dfrac{2}{3}$	$\dfrac{1}{3}$
Conditional		
2 unaffected sons	$\dfrac{1}{4}$	1
Joint	$\dfrac{1}{6}$	$\dfrac{1}{3}$

Example 3: Incorporating Unaffected Male Antecedents

This example is similar to that outlined in Example 2, but now the consultant, III4 in Figure 4.5, in addition to having two unaffected brothers, also has two unaffected maternal uncles. Intuitively, it is apparent that these two uncles make it less likely that the grandmother, I2, is a carrier, so that the risk for III4 will be less than that in Example 2. The precise risk is calculated by constructing a Bayesian table taking into account all possibilities (Table 4.5). This gives a posterior probability that II2 is a carrier of $(\mu/16 + \mu/4)/(\mu/16 + \mu/4 + \mu)$, which equals 5/21.

Therefore, the prior probability that III4 is a carrier equals 5/42, which is considerably less than the value of 1/6 obtained in Example 2. Note that the shortcut approach using a prior probability of 2/3 for II2 would have given the wrong answer in this example since it would not have taken into account the two unaffected maternal uncles.

From this Bayesian table it is also possible to establish the posterior probability that I2 is a carrier. This will be $(\mu/16)/(\mu/16 + \mu/4 + \mu)$, which equals 1/21. This can be used as a starting point if the daughter of I2, i.e., II5, is the consultand. Thus, the prior probability that II5 is a carrier equals 1/42.

Key Point 3

To incorporate information about male ancestors in the matrilineal line, a Bayesian table should be drawn up commencing with the common maternal female ancestor.

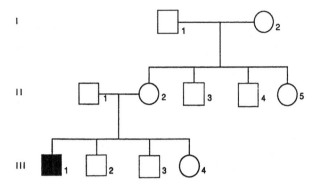

Figure 4.5. III4 is the consultand.

Table 4.5.

Probability	I2 Is a Carrier		I2 Is Not a Carrier	
Prior	4μ		$1 - 4\mu = 1$	
Conditional 2 unaffected sons	$\dfrac{1}{4}$		1	
II2	Carrier	Not a carrier	Carrier	Not a carrier
Prior	$\dfrac{1}{2}$	$\dfrac{1}{2}$	2μ	1
Conditional 1 affected son	$\dfrac{1}{2}$	μ	$\dfrac{1}{2}$	μ
2 unaffected sons	$\dfrac{1}{4}$	1	$\dfrac{1}{4}$	1
	$\mu/16$	$\mu^2/2$	$\mu/4$	μ

Example 4: Incorporating Unaffected Male Descendants

So far, we have considered those situations in which risks are modified by unaffected male siblings and matrilineal ancestors. Figure 4.6 shows a situation in which unaffected male descendants have to be considered. In this example, III1 is the consultand. Once again, a Bayesian table (Table 4.6) is constructed that incorporates all possible genotypes. From this table, it is apparent that the posterior probability that III1 is a carrier equals $(\mu/512)/(\mu/512 + \mu/128 + \mu/8 + \mu)$, which equals 1/581.

The value of this approach is further illustrated if III2 is the consultand. Now the posterior probability that II5 is a carrier is calculated, i.e., $\dfrac{\mu/512 + \mu/128}{\mu/512 + \mu/128 + \mu/8 + \mu}$, which equals 5/581.

This value is then halved to obtain the prior probability that III2 is a carrier, i.e., 5/1162.

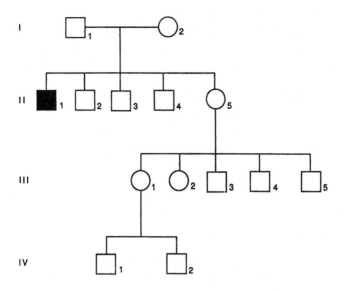

Figure 4.6. III1 is the consultand.

Table 4.6.

Probability	I2 Is a Carrier				I2 Is Not a Carrier			
Prior	4μ				$1-4\mu=1$			
Conditional								
1 affected son	$\frac{1}{2}$				μ			
3 unaffected sons	$\frac{1}{8}$				1			
II5	Carrier		Not carrier		Carrier		Not carrier	
Prior	$\frac{1}{2}$		$\frac{1}{2}$		2μ		1	
Conditional								
3 unaffected sons	$\frac{1}{8}$		1		$\frac{1}{8}$		1	
III1	C	NC	C	NC	C	NC	C	NC
Prior	$\frac{1}{2}$	$\frac{1}{2}$	2μ	1	$\frac{1}{2}$	$\frac{1}{2}$	2μ	1
Conditional								
2 unaffected sons	$\frac{1}{4}$	1	$\frac{1}{4}$	1	$\frac{1}{4}$	1	$\frac{1}{4}$	1
Joint	$\mu/512$	$\mu/128$	$\mu^2/16$	$\mu/8$	$\mu^2/32$	$\mu^2/8$	$\mu^2/2$	μ

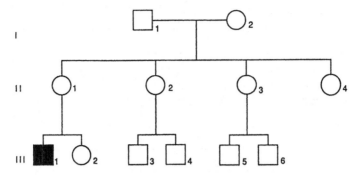

Figure 4.7. II4 and III2 are the consultands.

Example 5

This example is included to emphasize the importance of taking into account all unaffected males descended in the matrilineal line from females who could be carriers. In Figure 4.7 two consultands are considered, i.e., III2 and II4. Once again, a Bayesian table (Table 4.7) is constructed that incorporates all possible genotypes.

From this the posterior probability that I2 is a carrier equals $\frac{25\mu/64}{25\mu/64 + \mu + \mu}$, which reduces to 25/153. Similarly, the posterior probability that II1 is a carrier equals $\frac{25\mu/64 + \mu}{25\mu/64 + \mu + \mu}$, which reduces to 89/153. Therefore, for the consultands II4 and III2, prior probability values for being carriers are 25/306 and 89/306, respectively.

Note that if the four unaffected male cousins of the affected male had not been considered, the consultands II4 and III2 would have been given prior probability values for being carriers of 1/6 and 1/3, respectively. For II4 in particular, the four unaffected males have significantly reduced her prior probability of being a carrier.

We can use this example to demonstrate two useful points.

1. The conditional probability of two daughters, each with two unaffected sons, was stated as $[1/2 + (1/2 \times (1/2)^2)]^2$. This was derived as follows. A daughter

Table 4.7.

Probability	I2 Is a Carrier		I2 Is Not a Carrier	
Prior	4μ		$1 - 4\mu = 1$	
Conditional 2 daughters each with 2 unaffected sons	$\left[\frac{1}{2} + \left(\frac{1}{2} \times \left(\frac{1}{2}\right)^2\right)\right]^2$		1	
II1	Carrier	Not carrier	Carrier	Not carrier
Prior	$\frac{1}{2}$	$\frac{1}{2}$	2μ	1
Conditional 1 affected son	$\frac{1}{2}$	μ	$\frac{1}{2}$	μ
Joint	$25\mu/64$	$50\mu^2/64$	μ	μ

Table 4.8.

Probability	12 Is a Carrier			12 Is a Not a Carrier		
Prior	4μ			$1 - 4\mu = 1$		
Conditional III1 (1 affected son)	$\left(\dfrac{1}{2} \times \dfrac{1}{2}\right) + \left(\dfrac{1}{2} \times \mu\right)$ $= \dfrac{1}{4} + \mu/2$			$\left(2\mu \times \dfrac{1}{2}\right) + (1 \times \mu)$ $= 2\mu$		
II2 (2 unaffected sons)	$\left[\dfrac{1}{2} \times \left(\dfrac{1}{2}\right)^2\right] + \dfrac{1}{2} = \dfrac{5}{8}$			1		
II3	Carrier		Not carrier	Carrier		Not carrier
Prior	$\dfrac{1}{2}$		$\dfrac{1}{2}$	2μ		1
Conditional 2 unaffected sons	$\dfrac{1}{4}$		1	$\dfrac{1}{4}$		1
Joint	$5\mu/64 + 10\mu^2/64$		$5\mu/16 + 10\mu^2/16$	μ^2		2μ

Posterior probability that II3 is a carrier $= (5/64)\mu/((5/64)\mu + (5/16)\mu + 2\mu)$ (ignoring μ^2) $= 5/153$

with n unaffected sons yields a conditional probability of (1) the probability that she is not a carrier $= 1/2$ plus (2) the probability that she is a carrier $= 1/2$, multiplied by $(1/2)^n$, this latter value being the chance that n sons will be unaffected. This can be abbreviated as $1/2 + (1/2)(1/2)^n$ or $1/2 + (1/2)^{n+1}$. The contribution of a daughter with several unaffected grandsons will be almost as great as that of a single unaffected son. For example, a daughter with one, two, three, four, or five normal sons will contribute conditional probabilities of $3/4$, $5/8$, $9/16$, $17/32$, and $33/64$, respectively.

2. The way Table 4.7 has been constructed enables a carrier risk to be derived for I2 (and therefore also for II4) and II1. In its present form it does not enable a risk to be determined for II2 or II3. To achieve this, the table has to be redrawn as Table 4.8, in which a risk for II3 is obtained by considering her as the last individual under conditional probabilities. From Table 4.8 the carrier risk for II3 can be shown to be 5/153. An identical risk would be obtained for II2 using a table constructed to include II2 as the final individual to be included under conditional probabilities.

Key Point 4

Information about unaffected male descendants in the matrilineal female line should also be included. This is achieved by drawing up a Bayesian table commencing with the common matrilineal female ancestor and then including each relevant unaffected male as a conditional probability. A daughter with n unaffected sons contributes a conditional probability of $1/2 + (1/2)^{n+1}$.

Table 4.9

Probability	I2 Is a Carrier		I2 Is Not a Carrier	
Prior	4μ		$1 - 4\mu = 1$	
Conditional				
1 affected son	$\frac{1}{2}$		μ	
normal CK	$\frac{1}{3}$		0.95	
II2	Carrier	Not carrier	Carrier	Not carrier
Prior	$\frac{1}{2}$	$\frac{1}{2}$	2μ	1
Conditional				
normal CK	$\frac{1}{3}$	0.95	$\frac{1}{3}$	0.95
Joint	$\mu/9$	$0.95\mu/3$	$1.9\mu^2/3$	$\mu(0.95)^2$

CK, Creatine Kinase.

Example 6: Incorporating the Results of Carrier Tests

Results of carrier tests, which do not invariably show a clear distinction between the carrier and noncarrier states, can be included as conditional probabilities. For example, in Duchenne muscular dystrophy (DMD), approximately two out of three obligatory carriers show elevation of serum creatine kinase levels above the 95th percentile in the distribution obtained for women from the general population. Therefore, in Example 1 (Fig. 4.3), if both I2 and II2 have normal (i.e., below the 95th percentile) creatine kinase levels, this information can be incorporated in a Bayesian table (Table 4.9).

The posterior probabilities that I2 and II2 are carriers equal 0.32 and 0.08, respectively, considerably less than the values of 0.67 and 0.33 obtained if the normal creatine kinase results are not taken into account.

When the results of carrier tests show overlapping normal distributions in carriers and noncarriers, it is possible to calculate precise odds for carrier:noncarrier for any particular result. These odds can then be included as conditional probabilities, as outlined in this example. The method used for deriving these odds ratios is discussed in Appendix A.2.

Key Point 5

The results of carrier tests that show overlap between carriers and noncarriers can be included as conditional probabilities as long as the results of the various tests used are independent of each other, i.e., the parameters being measured are not interrelated.

4.4 Different Mutation Rates in Males and Females

In the examples considered so far, it has been assumed that the mutation rates in male and female germ cells are equal. While this is probably still a reasonable overall assumption for DMD when all cases are considered together (Müller et al., 1992), it has become clear that the male:female mutation ratio in many X-linked disorders is influenced by the nature of the underlying mutation (Table 4.10). Generally, the mutation rate in spermatogenesis has been shown to greatly exceed that in oogenesis, almost certainly because of the much greater opportunity for mitotic copy errors to occur in the male reproductive process.

If the mutation rate in males is much greater than that in females, then this increases the probability that the mother of an isolated case is a carrier. Thus, when counseling for a condition such as DMD, it is only reasonable to assume that the male:female mutation ratio is 1 ($\mu = v$) and that the prior probability that a woman is a carrier equals 4μ if no mutation studies have been undertaken. For example, if it has been shown that a boy who is an isolated case of DMD is negative on dystrophin deletion testing, so that he probably has an underlying point mutation, then the probability that his mother is a carrier is greater than $2/3$, as most point mutations will have originated in spermatogenesis in his maternal grandfather or great-grandfather.

When calculating risks in disorders in which it is known that male and female mutation rates are not equal, the first step is to determine the prior probability that any female is a carrier using the formula $P = 2\mu + 2v$ derived in Figure 4.1. For a disorder such as the Lesch-Nyhan syndrome, in which the male: female mutation rate is approximately 10:1 (i.e., $v = 10\mu$), the prior probability that any female is a carrier equals $2\mu + 2v = 2\mu + 20\mu = 22\mu$. This value can then be used in a standard Bayesian calculation, as shown in Example 7.

Table 4.10. Male:Female Mutation Ratio in X-Linked Disorders

Disorder	Male:Female Mutation Ratio	Reference
Duchenne muscular dystrophy		
All cases	1:1	Müller et al. (1992)
Deletions/duplications	0.3:1	
Point mutations	40:1	Grimm et al. (1994)
Hemophilia A		
All cases	3.6:1	
Deletions	<1:5	
Inversions	>10:1	
Point mutations	5–10:1	Becker et al. (1996)
Hemophilia B		
All cases	8.6:1	Green et al. (1999)
Lesch-Nyhan syndrome	10:1	Francke et al. (1976)
Myotubular myopathy	6.3:1	Herman et al. (2002)
Ornithine transcarbamylase deficiency	50:1	Tuchman et al. (1995)

Table 4.11.

Probability	Carrier	Not a Carrier
Prior	$2\mu(1+r)$	1
Conditional		
1 affected son	$\dfrac{1}{2}$	μ
Joint	$\overline{\mu(1+r)}$	$\overline{\mu}$

Posterior probability that the mother is a carrier (PC = x) equals $\mu(1+r)/$ $[\mu(1+r)+\mu]=(1+r)/(2+r)$. Therefore, $x=(1+r)/(2+r)$ and (by simple algebra) $r=(2x-1)/(1-x)$.

If the male:female mutation ratio is not known, but it has been established that the proportion of mothers of isolated cases who are carriers is greater or less than 2/3, then an estimate of the male:female mutation ratio ($v/\mu=r$) can be made as follows (Table 4.11). The prior probability that the mother is a carrier equals $2\mu+2v$, which equals $2\mu+2\mu r=2\mu(1+r)$, as $r=v/\mu$. As indicated in Table 4.11, the posterior probability that the mother is a carrier equals $(1+r)/(2+r)$ (Grimm et al., 1994). Using a little simple algebra, it can be shown that if the proportion of mothers of isolated cases shown to be carriers equals x, then the male:female mutation ratio, r, equals $(2x-1)/(1-x)$ (Flodman and Spence, 2003). Values for r, given different values of x, are indicated in Table 4.12. Note that these values are based on the assumption that the fitness of affected males equals zero. Calculations for disorders in which fitness is greater than zero are considered in the next section.

Table 4.12.   Relationship Between Proportion of Mothers of Isolated Cases Who Are Carriers and Male:Female Mutation Rate in X-Linked Disorders

Proportion of Mothers Who Are Carriers (= x in Table 4.11)	Male:Female Mutation Ratio (= r in Table 4.11)
0.5	Mutations occur only in female
0.55	0.22
0.6	0.5
0.65	0.86
0.67 (2/3)	1
0.7	1.33
0.75	2
0.8	3
0.85	4.67
0.9	8
0.95	18
1	Mutations occur only in male

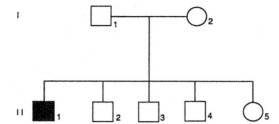

Figure 4.8. II5 is the consultand.

Table 4.13.

Probability	I2 Is a Carrier	I2 Is Not a Carrier
Prior	22μ	$1 - 22\mu = 1$
Conditional		
3 unaffected sons	$\dfrac{1}{8}$	1
1 affected son	$\dfrac{1}{2}$	μ
Joint	$11\mu/8$	μ

Example 7

In this example (Fig. 4.8), II5 is the consultand. She has one brother with a disorder such as the Lesch-Nyhan syndrome in which $v = 10\mu$. She also has three unaffected brothers. The prior probability that II5 is a carrier is calculated by determining the posterior probability that her mother, I2, is a carrier in the usual way (Table 4.13).

The posterior probability that I2 is a carrier equals $(11\mu/8)/(11\mu/8 + \mu)$, which equals 11/19, so that the prior probability that II5 is a carrier equals 11/38.

Mutation Occurs Only in Male Germ Cells

If mutation occurs exclusively in male germ cells, then all mothers of isolated cases must be carriers. Thus, there will be a prior probability of 1/2 that the sister of an isolated case will be a carrier, regardless of how many unaffected brothers she has, so that risks for female descendants can be calculated as outlined in previous examples.

However, the estimation of risks for antecedent females in the matrilineal line is more difficult. By using the Adam and Eve model outlined in Figure 4.1, it can be shown that the prior probability that any female is a carrier of an X-linked recessive disorder, in which biological fitness equals zero and mutation (v) occurs only in male germ cells, equals $2v$. Thus, when constructing a Bayesian table that incorporates all possibilities, this value of $2v$ should be used as the prior probability that the common female ancestor of the proband and consultand is a carrier. Furthermore, it should be remembered that if a female is not a carrier, then there is zero probability that she can

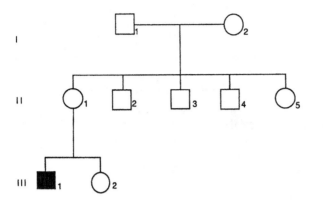

Figure 4.9. II5 is the
consultand.

Table 4.14.

Probability	I2 Is a Carrier		I2 Is Not a Carrier	
Prior	$2v$		$1 - 2v = 1$	
Conditional				
3 unaffected sons	$\dfrac{1}{8}$		1	
II1	Carrier	Not carrier	Carrier	Not carrier
Prior	$\dfrac{1}{2}$	$\dfrac{1}{2}$	v	1
Conditional				
1 affected son	$\dfrac{1}{2}$	0	$\dfrac{1}{2}$	0
Joint	$v/16$	0	$v/2$	0

have an affected son, since mutation occurs only in male germ cells and obviously a son can only inherit an X chromosome from his mother.

Example 8

In this example (Fig. 4.9) the consultand is II5. As in previous examples, her prior probability of being a carrier is determined by calculating the posterior probability that her mother is a carrier and then halving this value (Table 4.14).

The posterior probability that I2 is a carrier equals $(v/16)/(v/16 + v/2)$, which equals 1/9, so that the prior probability that II5 is a carrier equals 1/18.

Mutation Occurs Only in Female Germ Cells

If mutation occurs only in female germ cells, and μ equals the mutation rate, then by using the Adam and Eve model once more, it can be shown that the prior probability that any female is a carrier of a particular X-linked recessive disorder equals 2μ. This allows risks for antecedent and descendant females to be calculated as illustrated in the two following examples.

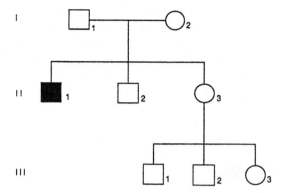

Figure 4.10. III3 is the consultand.

Example 9

In this example (Fig. 4.10) III3 is the consultand. The prior probability that she is a carrier is determined as usual by calculating the posterior probability that her mother, II3, is a carrier and then halving this result (Table 4.15).

The posterior probability that II3 is a carrier equals $(\mu/16)/(\mu/16 + \mu/4 + \mu)$, which equals 1/21, so that the prior probability that III3 is a carrier equals 1/42.

Key Point 6

If the mutation rates differ in males and females, the prior probability that a female is a carrier can be calculated from the formula

$$C = 2\mu + 2v$$

where μ is the mutation rate in females and v is the mutation rate in males.

Table 4.15.

Probability	I2 Is a Carrier		I2 Is Not a Carrier	
Prior	2μ		$1 - 2\mu = 1$	
Conditional				
1 affected son	$\dfrac{1}{2}$		μ	
1 unaffected son	$\dfrac{1}{2}$		1	
II3	Carrier	Not carrier	Carrier	Not carrier
Prior	$\dfrac{1}{2}$	$\dfrac{1}{2}$	μ	1
Conditional sons				
2 unaffected sons	$\dfrac{1}{4}$	1	$\dfrac{1}{4}$	1
Joint	$\mu/16$	$\mu/4$	$\mu^2/4$	μ

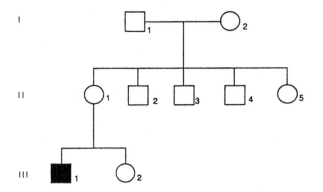

Figure 4.11. II5 is the consultand.

Table 4.16.

Probability	I2 Is a Carrier		I2 Is Not a Carrier	
Prior	2μ		$1 - 2\mu = 1$	
Conditional 3 unaffected sons	$\frac{1}{8}$		1	
III1	Carrier	Not carrier	Carrier	Not carrier
Prior	$\frac{1}{2}$	$\frac{1}{2}$	μ	1
Conditional 1 affected son	$\frac{1}{2}$	μ	$\frac{1}{2}$	μ
Joint	$\mu/16$	$\mu^2/8$	$\mu/2$	μ

Example 10

In this example (Fig. 4.11) II5 is the consultand. The calculation is as shown in Table 4.16. The posterior probability that I2 is a carrier equals $(\mu/16)/(\mu/16 + \mu/2 + \mu)$, which equals 1/25, and the prior probability that II5 is a carrier equals 1/50.

4.5 Biological Fitness Is Greater Than Zero

Biological (genetic) fitness refers to the capacity to reproduce and have healthy children. It is usually expressed as a proportion of 1. Thus, if fitness in a certain X-linked recessive disorder is said to be 0.5, this implies that, on average, affected males have only half as many offspring as their unaffected male siblings or healthy members of the general population.

    In all of the examples considered so far, it has been assumed that biological fitness equals zero, so that the probability that an affected male will transmit his abnormal gene is zero. However, in many X-linked recessive disorders fitness is only mildly impaired, and this will have a major influence when estimating the prior probability that any female is a carrier, since it becomes possible that she may have inherited the mutant gene from her affected father.

Therefore, the prior probability that any female is a carrier will be greater than the value of $2\mu + 2v$ derived earlier in this chapter when biological fitness was assumed to be zero. Various approaches to the derivation of this new value for the prior probability that any female is a carrier have been described (Grimm, 1984; Haldane, 1947). The simplest explanation, which has the major advantage of being reasonably comprehensible, is as follows.

A female can be a carrier of an X-linked recessive disorder for any one of three reasons:

1. Her mother may be a carrier (*PM*).
2. A new mutation may occur in the female (μ) or male (v) germ cell.
3. Her father may be affected (*PI*).

Thus, the probability (*PF*) that a female is a carrier can be written as

$$PF = 1/2\,PM + \mu + v + f\,PI \tag{1}$$

where *f* equals the biological fitness of affected males.

A male can be affected for one of two reasons:

1. His mother may be a carrier (*PM*).
2. A new mutation may occur in the female germ cell (μ).

This can be written as

$$PI = 1/2\,PM + \mu \tag{2}$$

If the disease under consideration is in genetic equilibrium, then the prior probability that a mother is a carrier will equal the prior probability that her daughter is a carrier, i.e., *PF = PM*. Substituting this, and equation (2) into equation (1), gives

$$PF = 1/2\,PF + \mu + v + f(1/2\,PF + \mu) \tag{3}$$

By simple algebra this reduces to

$$PF = \frac{2\mu + 2v + 2\mu f}{1 - f} \tag{4}$$

and if mutation rates in male and female germ cells are equal, then

$$PF = \frac{4\mu + 2\mu f}{1 - f} \tag{5}$$

Example 11

In the pedigree in Figure 4.12, there is an isolated case of Becker muscular dystrophy (BMD), an X-linked recessive disorder in which fitness has been estimated to be approximately 0.7 (Emery, 1997) and in which, by analogy with the allelic DMD, the overall male:female mutation rate is probably close to 1. From equation (5) it can be calculated that the prior probability that any female is a carrier equals 18μ.

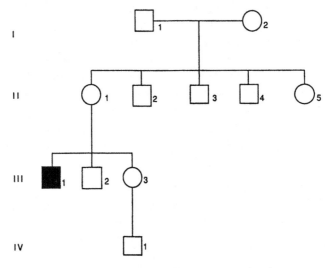

Figure 4.12. II5 and III3 are the consultands.

In this example, it is assumed that there are two consultands, II5 and III3. As in previous examples, a table is constructed that incorporates all possible genotypes (Table 4.17).

The posterior probability that I2 is a carrier equals

$$\frac{9\mu/128 + 9\mu/64}{9\mu/128 + 9\mu/64 + \mu/8 + \mu/4 + \mu}$$

Table 4.17.

Probability	I2 Is a Carrier				I2 Is Not a Carrier			
Prior	18μ				$1 - 18\mu = 1$			
Conditional 3 unaffected sons	$\dfrac{1}{8}$				1			
II1	Carrier		Not carrier		Carrier		Not carrier	
Prior	$\dfrac{1}{2}$		$\dfrac{1}{2}$		2μ		1	
Conditional 1 affected son	$\dfrac{1}{2}$		μ		$\dfrac{1}{2}$		μ	
1 unaffected son	$\dfrac{1}{2}$		1		$\dfrac{1}{2}$		1	
III3	C	NC	C	NC	C	NC	C	NC
Prior	$\dfrac{1}{2}$	$\dfrac{1}{2}$	2μ	1	$\dfrac{1}{2}$	$\dfrac{1}{2}$	2μ	1
Conditional 1 unaffected son	$\dfrac{1}{2}$	1	$\dfrac{1}{2}$	1	$\dfrac{1}{2}$	1	$\dfrac{1}{2}$	1
Joint	$9\mu/128$	$9\mu/64$	$9\mu^3/8$	$9\mu^2/8$	$\mu/8$	$\mu/4$	μ^2	μ

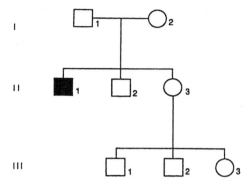

Figure 4.13. III3 is the consultand.

which equals 27/203. Therefore, the prior probability that II5 is a carrier equals 27/406. Similarly, the posterior probability that III3 is a carrier equals

$$\frac{9\mu/128 + \mu/8}{9\mu/128 + 9\mu/64 + \mu/8 + \mu/4 + \mu}$$

which equals 25/203.

Example 12

In this example (Fig. 4.13) the family pedigree reveals a single case of hemophilia B, for which the overall mutation rate in males (v) is thought to be approximately 8 to 10 times greater than that in females (μ). Various estimates of the biological fitness of affected males have been made, ranging from 0.3 to 0.7. In this example a value of 0.5 is assumed.

If $f = 0.5$ and $v = 10\mu$, then from equation (4) it can be calculated that there is a prior probability of 46μ that any female is a carrier. Using this as the prior probability that I2 is a carrier, the calculation of the prior probability that the consultand, III3, is a carrier proceeds as in Table 4.18.

The posterior probability that II3 is a carrier equals

$$\frac{23\mu/16}{23\mu/16 + 23\mu/4 + \mu}$$

which equals 23/131, and the prior probability that the consultant, III3, is a carrier equals 23/262.

In Examples 11 and 12 (Figs. 4.12 and 4.13), if it is known that the fathers of individuals I2 in each pedigree were not affected, then the prior probability for each of these women being a carrier will be reduced. In Example 11, the prior probability that I2 is a carrier becomes 11μ instead of 18μ, the value of 11μ being the sum of 9μ (half of the probability that her mother is a carrier) plus 2μ (the probability of a mutation having occurred on either the maternally or paternally derived X chromosome). In example 12, the prior probability that I2 is a carrier becomes 34μ, this being the sum of 23μ (half of the probability that her mother is a

Table 4.18.

Probability	I2 Is a Carrier		I2 Is Not a Carrier	
Prior	46μ		$1 - 46\mu = 1$	
Conditional				
1 affected son	$\dfrac{1}{2}$		μ	
1 unaffected son	$\dfrac{1}{2}$		1	
II3	Carrier	Not carrier	Carrier	Not carrier
Prior	$\dfrac{1}{2}$	$\dfrac{1}{2}$	$\mu + v = 11\mu$	1
Conditional				
2 unaffected sons	$\dfrac{1}{4}$	1	$\dfrac{1}{4}$	1
Joint	$23\mu/16$	$23\mu/4$	$11\mu^2/4$	μ

carrier), plus μ (the probability that a mutation occurred on the maternally derived X chromosome) plus v ($=10\mu$) (the probability that a mutation occurred on the paternally derived X chromosome).

Key Point 7

If the biological fitness in affected males is greater than zero, the prior probability that a female is a carrier (PF) can be calculated from the formula

$$PF = \frac{4\mu + 2\mu f}{1 - f}$$

where μ is the mutation rate in females and f is the genetic fitness of affected males.

4.6 Case Scenario

Figure 4.14 shows a pedigree in which two males, III1 and IV1, have had severe unexplained learning difficulties. Fragile X mutation analysis in IV1 gave a normal result. On the basis of their relationship through an unaffected female, the reasonable conclusion is reached that these males probably had severe nonspecific X-linked mental retardation. Two female relatives, IV4 and V4, wish to know the risk that they could be carriers.

The probability that V4 is a carrier can be determined relatively easily by drawing up a simple Bayesian table (Table 4.19) starting with individual IV2, for whom the prior probability for being a carrier is 1/2. The posterior probability that IV2 is a carrier equals 5/37, so that the prior probability that her daughter, V4, is a carrier equals 5/74, or approximately 1 in 15. Note that taking into account the two unaffected sons and two unaffected grandsons of IV2 has markedly reduced the carrier risk for V4 from 1 in 4 to this value of 1 in 15.

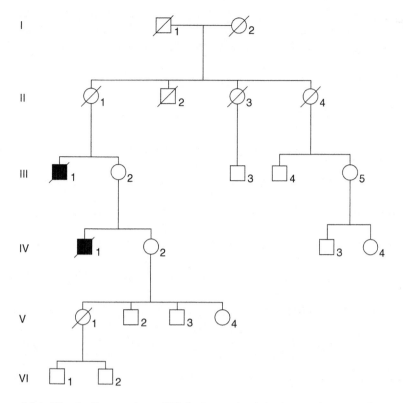

Figure 4.14. The family tree shows X-linked recessive inheritance of nonspecific mental retardation.

Table 4.19   (see Case Scenario)

Probability	IV2 Is a Carrier	IV2 Is Not a Carrier
Prior	$\dfrac{1}{2}$	$\dfrac{1}{2}$
Conditional		
2 unaffected sons	$\dfrac{1}{4}$	1
daughter with 2 unaffected sons	$\dfrac{5}{8}$	1
Joint	$\dfrac{5}{64}$	$\dfrac{1}{2}$

Posterior probability that IV2 is a carrier equals $\dfrac{5}{64} \Big/ \left(\dfrac{5}{64} + \dfrac{1}{2}\right) = 5/37$. Therefore, the prior probability that V4 is a carrier equals $5/74$ (approximately 1 in 15).

Table 4.20.

Probability	I2 Is a Carrier				I2 Is Not a Carrier			
Prior	4μ				1			
Conditional								
1 unaffected son	$\frac{1}{2}$				1			
daughter with 1 son	$\frac{3}{4}$				1			
carrier daughter (III1)	$\frac{1}{2}$				2μ			
II4	C		NC		C		NC	
Prior	$\frac{1}{2}$		$\frac{1}{2}$		2μ		1	
Conditional	$\frac{1}{2}$		1		$\frac{1}{2}$		1	
III5	C	NC	C	NC	C	NC	C	NC
Prior	$\frac{1}{2}$	$\frac{1}{2}$	2μ	1	$\frac{1}{2}$	$\frac{1}{2}$	2μ	1
Conditional								
1 unaffected son	$\frac{1}{2}$	1	$\frac{1}{2}$	1	$\frac{1}{2}$	1	$\frac{1}{2}$	1
Joint	$3\mu/64$	$3\mu/32$	$3\mu^2/8$	$3\mu/8$	$\mu^2/2$	μ^2	$2\mu^2$	2μ

Posterior probability that III5 is a carrier equals $3/64(3/64 + 3/32 + 3/8 + 2) = 3/161$. Therefore, the prior probability that IV4 is a carrier equals $3/322$, i.e., <1%.

Determining the carrier risk for IV4 is more difficult. It is assumed that male and female mutation rates are equal and that the genetic fitness of affected males is zero. This allows a value of 4μ to be assigned as the prior probability that I2 was a carrier. A Bayesian table is then constructed (Table 4.20) in which it is assumed that II1 was a carrier, as she transmitted mutant alleles to both of her children, III1 and III2. The alternative possibility is that II1 was a germline mosaic, as discussed in Chapter 6. Thus, this assumption of carrier status in II1 gives a maximum estimate of risk for collateral relatives such as II4 and her descendants. Table 4.20 indicates that the posterior probability that III5 is a carrier equals 3/161, so that the prior probability that IV4 is a carrier equals 3/322, i.e., less than 1%.

Further Reading

Flodman, P. and Hodge, S.E. (2002). Determining complex genetic risks by computer. *Journal of Genetic Counseling*. **11**, 213–230.

Flodman, P. and Hodge, S.E. (2003). Sex-specific mutation rates for X-linked disorders: estimation and application. *Human Heredity*, **55**, 51–55.

Murphy, E.A. and Chase, G.A. (1975). *Principles of genetic counseling*. Year Book Medical Publishers, Chicago.

Murphy, E.A. and Mutalik, G.S. (1969). The application of Bayesian methods in genetic counseling. *Human Heredity*, **19**, 126–151.

5

The Use of Linked
DNA Markers

Developments in molecular genetics have greatly enhanced the diagnostic repertoire of the clinical geneticist. If a specific pathogenic mutation can be identified in a family, then carrier detection, preclinical detection, and prenatal diagnosis become relatively straightforward. However, situations can still arise in which a specific mutation cannot be identified, possibly because a sample cannot be obtained from an affected individual or because the relevant gene has not been isolated even though the disease has been mapped to a particular chromosome region. In both of these situations, a compromise solution involves the use of polymorphic DNA marker loci that have been shown to be genetically linked to the disorder in question. Genetic linkage is a complex subject, and the use of linked DNA markers can generate some very difficult calculations. Sometimes these issues are best resolved with the help of one of the computer packages that have been developed (Lathrop and Lalouel, 1984). Simple calculations can usually be managed using pencil and paper, and even in situations where this is not possible, it is useful to understand the basic principles involved so that an attempt can be made to assess whether the answer provided by the computer program is plausible. This chapter offers an approach to the solution of some of the less complex linkage calculations that can be carried out on the back of the proverbial envelope (sometimes a rather large envelope is needed!).

5.1 Basic Principles of Genetic Linkage

Two loci are said to show *genetic linkage* if alleles at these loci segregate together more often than would be expected by chance, i.e., the two loci are so close together on the same chromosome (*syntenic*) that it is unlikely that they will be separated by a crossover event at meiosis. The likelihood that any two alleles at two randomly selected loci will be inherited together is 0.5. If alleles at two loci are inherited together significantly more often than in 50% of meioses, then these loci are linked. Alleles at linked loci on the same chromosome are said to be in *coupling*, whereas those on opposite homologous chromosomes are said to be in *repulsion*. This is known as the linkage *phase*.

The *recombination fraction* (θ) is an indication of the genetic distance between two loci; more precisely, it is a measure of the likelihood of recombination occurring between them. The closer together the two loci are, the smaller the recombination fraction. If two loci are not linked, then θ equals 0.5, as on average, genes at unlinked loci will segregate together in 50% of all meioses. If θ equals less than 0.5, then the loci are linked. For example, if θ equals 0.05, then alleles in coupling at these loci will be inherited together during meiosis 19 times out of 20.

The term *polymorphic DNA marker* refers to variation, usually harmless, in DNA at a specific locus, which can be identified using one of a number of standard laboratory techniques. A polymorphic DNA marker can consist of (1) a restriction fragment length polymorphism (RFLP) generated by variation in a nucleotide that occurs within the recognition sequence of a restriction enzyme, (2) a variable number tandem repeat (VNTR) resulting from the presence of a variable number of tandem repeats of a short DNA sequence, (3) a *microsatellite*, also known as a *CA repeat*, or (4) a single nucleotide polymorphism (SNP). VNTRs, microsatellites, and SNPs are particularly useful DNA markers, as they are highly polymorphic, easily demonstrated, and inherited in a Mendelian codominant fashion. If it is possible to identify a polymorphic DNA marker locus that is linked to a disease locus, then this can be used to modify risks to close family members, as illustrated in the examples that follow later in this chapter.

Lod scores are a mathematic device often used to confirm or refute linkage of two or more loci. A lod score (equals log of the odds) is calculated as the logarithm to the base 10 of the ratio of the likelihood that two loci are linked for a given value of θ to the likelihood that they are not linked, i.e.,

$$\log_{10} \frac{\text{likelihood of linkage for a particular value of } \theta}{\text{likelihood that loci are unlinked (i.e., } \theta = 0.5)}$$

The underlying principle can be demonstrated using the family shown in Figure 5.1. Simple inspection indicates that all affected individuals in the third generation have inherited allele A from their father, whereas all unaffected individuals have inherited allele B. This obviously suggests that allele A is linked to the disease locus. To quantify this, a lod score is calculated. If the disease and marker loci are linked, then in individual II1 the disease locus must be in coupling with marker A, as both of these alleles have been inherited from the affected father in the first generation. If the two loci are so tightly linked that recombination between them rarely if ever occurs (i.e., θ equals 0), then the probability of observing the pattern of segregation seen in Figure 5.1 will be $(1 - \theta)^{10}$, which equals 1. If the loci are not linked, so that θ equals 0.5, then the likelihood of observing cosegregation of the disease and marker A in all 10 children of the third generation will equal $(1/2)^{10}$, which equals 1/1024. The lod score for this family given a value of $\theta = 0$ therefore equals the log base 10 of 1 divided by 1/1024, which equals 3.0103.

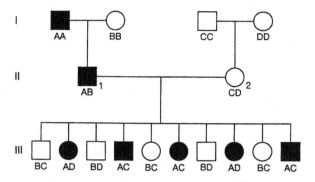

Figure 5.1. A, B, C, and D are allelic polymorphic markers. It is apparent that there has been no recombination between the marker locus and the disease locus in the 10 offspring of II1. Since the linkage phase in II1 is known (the disease gene must be in coupling with marker A), it is possible to conclude that linkage with a recombination fraction of zero is $1^{10}/0.5^{10} = 1024$ times more probable than no linkage. See the text for full discussion.

Generally, a lod score of 3 or greater is accepted as confirmation of linkage. This suggests odds of 1000 to 1 in favor of linkage, but in fact, the true probability is roughly 20 to 1 since there is a prior probability of approximately 50 to 1 that any two randomly selected genetic loci will not be linked.

This discussion of lod scores and genetic linkage has been included to provide a background for and a basic understanding of the principles involved in demonstrating linkage and calculating the recombination fraction. The important point to remember is that the recombination fraction (θ) indicates the probability that two alleles at linked loci on the same chromosome (i.e., in coupling) will be separated by a recombination event during meiosis. This will be a recurring theme in the examples that follow.

Key Point 1

Two loci are linked if they are positioned close to each other so that they are inherited together during more than 50% of meioses. Linked alleles on the same chromosome are in coupling; those on opposite chromosomes are in repulsion. The recombination fraction (θ) indicates the proportion of meioses during which alleles at linked loci will be separated by recombination.

5.2 Autosomal Dominant Inheritance

Example 1—Phase Known

A and B in Figure 5.2 represent allelic markers at a locus closely linked to the disease locus. Study of the pedigree indicates that in II2 the disease gene must be in coupling with marker A, as both the disease and this marker must have been inherited from I1. Note that this does not automatically imply that the disease gene

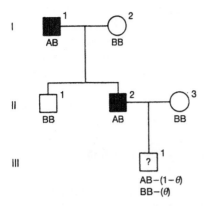

Figure 5.2. The disease gene in II2 must be in coupling with marker A. Thus, the risk for III1 if he inherits marker A will be $1 - \theta$ or θ if marker B is inherited.

in I1 is on the same chromosome as marker A, since a crossover could have occurred at meiosis in the formation of the gamete that resulted in II2.

Knowing that the disease is in coupling with marker A in II2 enables the disease status for III1 to be predicted. If he inherits the A marker, then the likelihood that he will be affected equals $1 - \theta$, i.e., he will be affected unless a crossover occurs at paternal meiosis. Similarly, the likelihood that he will not be affected equals θ. For a value of $\theta = 0.05$, the probability that III1 will be affected if he inherits marker A equals 0.95, and if he inherits marker B it equals 0.05.

Example 2: Phase unknown

In this example (Fig. 5.3) the phase is known in II1, but not in I1 for the reason already explained in Example 1. Therefore, in assessing the risk to II2, the calculation has to take into account the possibility that the disease in I1 is in coupling with either A or B. This is achieved using Bayes' theorem, in which prior information and observed (conditional) information are combined to derive posterior or relative probabilities for each event (Table 5.1). Bayes' theorem and its application in risk calculation are discussed at length elsewhere in Chapter 1.

The posterior probability that the disease in I1 is in coupling with A equals $(1-\theta)/2/[(1-\theta)/2 + \theta/2]$, which equals $1-\theta$. Similarly, the posterior probability that the disease in I1 is in coupling with B equals θ.

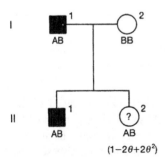

Figure 5.3. The phase for I1 is not known, but information about its likelihood can be obtained from II1, as indicated in the text. This then enables the risk for II2 to be calculated.

Table 5.1.

Probability	Disease in I1 in Coupling with A	Disease in I1 in Coupling with B
Prior	$\dfrac{1}{2}$	$\dfrac{1}{2}$
Conditional		
I11, who is affected, has inherited A	$1 - \theta$	θ
Joint	$\dfrac{1}{2}(1 - \theta)$	$\dfrac{1}{2}\theta$

For II2 in Figure 5.3, the calculation proceeds as follows. The probability that this individual has the disease gene, given that she has inherited marker A, equals the sum of

1. the probability that the disease in I1 is in coupling with A $(1-\theta)$ multiplied by $1-\theta$ i.e., $(1-\theta)^2$ plus
2. the probability that the disease in I1 is in coupling with B(θ) multiplied by (θ), i.e., θ^2. This summates to $1 - 2\theta + 2\theta^2$. In this situation there is therefore a predictive error of approximately 2θ, i.e., double that in Example 1, in which the linkage phase was known with certainty.

Readers who are particularly comfortable with the concept and principles of linkage might be able to deduce this answer of $1 - 2\theta + 2\theta^2$ using a little simple logic. Basically, the probability that II2 will be affected if she inherits A equals 1 minus (1) the probability that the disease allele in I1 is in coupling with A and is transmitted to II1 $(1 - \theta)$ but not to II2 (θ)—i.e., $(1 - \theta)\theta = \theta - \theta^2$, minus (2) the probability that the disease allele in I1 is in coupling with B and is transmitted to II1 (θ) but not to II2 $(1 - \theta)$—i.e., $\theta(1 - \theta) = \theta - \theta^2$. This gives a total of $1 - 2\theta + 2\theta^2$, as derived above.

Key Point 2

When the linkage phase in the transmitting parent is known, inheritance of the high-risk linked marker conveys a predictive error of θ, i.e., the probability that a crossover will occur. When the linkage phase in the transmitting parent is not known, inheritance of the high-risk linked marker conveys a predictive error of approximately 2θ because of the greater number of recombination events that could have occurred.

Example 3: Prenatal Exclusion Diagnosis

In Figure 5.4, II1 has not yet reached the age of onset of a serious late-onset neurological disorder. As her affected mother is homozygous for the linked disease marker, there is no means of predicting the disease status for II1. However, if she so wished, it would be possible to test her pregnancy to see if the fetus has inherited

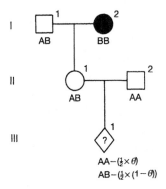

Figure 5.4. There is a probability of 0.5 that the B marker in II1 is in coupling with the disease gene. Thus, there will be a probability of $0.5 \times (1 - \theta)$ that any child of II1 inheriting the B marker will also inherit the disease gene.

marker A from its grandfather or marker B from its affected grandmother. Marker A would convey a risk of $1/2 \times \theta$ to the fetus (i.e., very low), whereas marker B would convey a risk of $1/2 \times (1 - \theta)$, which would be close to 50%. The detection of marker A in the fetus would therefore indicate that the risk is very low, i.e., *prenatal exclusion.*

5.3 Autosomal Recessive Inheritance

Example 4: Information from One Child

The first child of healthy parents in Figure 5.5 has an autosomal recessive disorder, and prenatal diagnosis is available using a closely linked marker with alleles A and B. Calculation of the probability that II2 will be affected given different genotypes AA, AB, and BB has to take into consideration the posterior probabilities for the linkage phase in the parents conditional upon information provided by II1, who is affected and has an AA marker genotype. These posterior probabilities are calculated as shown in Table 5.2.

From this table the posterior probability for each combination of parental genotypes can be calculated in the usual way and shown to be

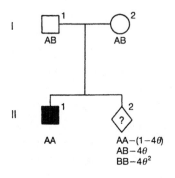

Figure 5.5. Approximate values for the likelihood that II2 will be affected given different marker genotypes are indicated.

Table 5.2. Linkage Phase of Disease Gene in Father (F) and Mother (M)

Probability	F(A)M(A)	F(A)M(B)	F(B)M(A)	F(B)M(B)
Prior	$\dfrac{1}{4}$	$\dfrac{1}{4}$	$\dfrac{1}{4}$	$\dfrac{1}{4}$
Conditional				
II1 has AA	$(1-\theta)^2$	$(1-\theta)\theta$	$\theta(1-\theta)$	θ^2
Joint	$\dfrac{1}{4}(1-\theta)^2$	$\dfrac{1}{4}(1-\theta)\theta$	$\dfrac{1}{4}\theta(1-\theta)$	$\dfrac{1}{4}\theta^2$

Father A: Mother A—$(1-\theta)^2$
Father A: Mother B—$(1-\theta)\theta$
Father B: Mother A—$\theta(1-\theta)$
Father B: Mother B—θ^2

Using this information, the probability that the fetus (II2) will be affected given different marker genotypes is determined as follows.

1. Fetus (II2) has an AA genotype. The overall probability that the fetus will be affected given an AA genotype will be the sum of
   a. the probability if the disease gene is in coupling with A in both parents, i.e., $(1-\theta)^2 \times (1-\theta)^2$, plus
   b. the probability if the disease gene is in coupling with A in the father and B in the mother, i.e., $(1-\theta)\theta \times (1-\theta)\theta$, plus
   c. the probability if the disease gene is in coupling with B in the father and A in the mother, i.e., $\theta(1-\theta) \times \theta(1-\theta)$, plus
   d. the probability if the disease gene is in coupling with B in both parents, i.e., $\theta^2 \times \theta^2$. This summates to $(1-\theta)^4 + 2\theta^2(1-\theta)^2 + \theta^4$, which equals $1 - 4\theta + 8\theta^2 - 8\theta^3 + 4\theta^4$.
2. Fetus (II2) has a BB genotype. The overall probability that the fetus will be affected given a BB genotype will be the sum of
   a. the probability if the disease gene is in coupling with A in both parents, i.e., $(1-\theta)^2 \times \theta^2$, plus
   b. the probability if the disease gene is in coupling with A in the father and B in the mother, i.e., $(1-\theta)\theta \times \theta(1-\theta)$ plus
   c. the probability if the disease gene is in coupling with B in the father and A in the mother, i.e., $\theta(1-\theta) \times (1-\theta)\theta$ plus
   d. the probability if the disease gene is in coupling with B in both parents, i.e., $\theta^2 \times (1-\theta)^2$. This summates to $4\theta^2(1-\theta)^2$, which equals $4\theta^2 - 8\theta^3 + 4\theta^4$.
3. Fetus (II2) has an AB genotype. In this situation, the fetus could have inherited A from the father and B from the mother or vice versa. If it is assumed that the A has come from the father and the B from the mother, then the overall probability that the fetus will be affected will be the sum of
   a. the probability if the disease gene is in coupling with A in both parents, i.e., $(1-\theta)^2 \times (1-\theta)\theta$, plus
   b. the probability if the disease gene is in coupling with A in the father and B in the mother, i.e., $(1-\theta)\theta \times (1-\theta)^2$, plus

c. the probability if the disease gene is in coupling with B in the father and A in the mother, i.e., $\theta(1 - \theta) \times \theta^2$, plus

d. the probability if the disease gene is in coupling with B in both parents, i.e., $\theta^2 \times \theta(1 - \theta)$.

This summates to $2\theta(1 - \theta)^3 + 2\theta^3(1 - \theta)$, which equals $2\theta - 6\theta^2 + 8\theta^3 - 4\theta^4$. An identical result will be obtained if the fetus has inherited A from the mother and B from the father. Thus, whichever way the AB genotype has been derived, it conveys a probability of $2\theta - 6\theta^2 + 8\theta^3 - 4\theta^4$ for being affected, giving a total of $4\theta - 12\theta^2 + 16\theta^3 - 8\theta^4$.

Since θ is likely to be a very small number (i.e., less than 0.01 for most of the linked markers currently used in prenatal diagnosis), reasonable approximations for the probability that the fetus will be affected are

Genotype AA—$1–4\theta$
Genotype AB/BA—4θ
Genotype BB—$4\theta^2$

Key Point 3

In autosomal recessive inheritance when the parental linkage phases are not known with certainty, there are four opportunities for a recombination event to occur, leading to a predictive error of approximately 4θ if a fetus inherits the same markers as its affected sibling.

Example 5: Information from Two Children

Now the healthy parents have two affected children and, fortunately, they show concordance for the linked marker genotypes. If they were totally discordant, so that II1 had an AA genotype and II2 a BB genotype, then the family would not be *informative* and prenatal diagnosis could not be offered. If they were partially discordant, so that II1 had an AA genotype and II2 an AB genotype, then the family would be partially informative in that a fetus inheriting a BB genotype would be at low risk but at relatively high risk for each of the other two genotypes.

In these situations, the precise calculations become very complex. The example illustrated in Figure 5.6 shall be calculated in full. First of all, it is necessary to establish the probability that markers A and B are in coupling with the disease in the parents I1 and I2. This is done as shown in Table 5.3.

The posterior probability that the disease gene is in coupling with marker A in both parents equals

$$\frac{\frac{1}{4}(1 - \theta)^4}{\frac{1}{4}(1 - \theta)^4 + \frac{1}{2}\theta^2(1 - \theta)^2 + \frac{1}{4}\theta^4}$$

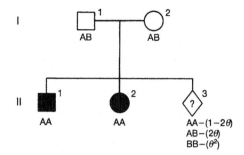

Figure 5.6. Approximate values for the likelihood that II3 will be affected given different marker genotypes are indicated, based on the assumption that concordant linkage information from the two affected children allows the linkage phase in the parents to be assumed.

which reduces to

$$\frac{1 - 4\theta + 6\theta^2 - 4\theta^3 + \theta^4}{1 - 4\theta + 8\theta^2 - 8\theta^3 + 4\theta^4} \tag{1}$$

By the same process, it can be shown that the posterior probabilities for the other possible disease gene linkage phases are

$$F(A):\, M(B) \qquad \frac{\theta^2 - 2\theta^3 + \theta^4}{1 - 4\theta + 8\theta^2 - 8\theta^3 + 4\theta^4} \tag{2}$$

$$F(B):\, M(A) \qquad \frac{\theta^2 - 2\theta^3 + \theta^4}{1 - 4\theta + 8\theta^2 - 8\theta^3 + 4\theta^4} \tag{3}$$

$$F(B):\, M(B) \qquad \frac{\theta^4}{1 - 4\theta + 8\theta^2 - 8\theta^3 + 4\theta^4} \tag{4}$$

The probability that II3 will be affected given different genotypes AA, AB, and BB can now be calculated as in Example 4. If the fetus (II3) inherits an AA genotype, the probability that it will be affected equals the sum of

a. $(1) \times (1 - \theta)^2$ plus
b. $(2) \times (1 - \theta)\theta$ plus
c. $(3) \times \theta(1 - \theta)$ plus
d. $(4) \times \theta^2$

Table 5.3. Linkage Phase of Disease Gene in Father (F) and Mother (M)

Probability	F(A)M(A)	F(A)M(B)	F(B)M(A)	F(B)M(B)
Prior	$\dfrac{1}{4}$	$\dfrac{1}{4}$	$\dfrac{1}{4}$	$\dfrac{1}{4}$
Conditional				
II1 (AA)	$(1 - \theta)^2$	$(1 - \theta)\theta$	$\theta(1 - \theta)$	θ^2
II2 (AA)	$(1 - \theta)^2$	$(1 - \theta)\theta$	$\theta(1 - \theta)$	θ^2
Joint	$\dfrac{1}{4}(1 - \theta)^4$	$\dfrac{1}{4}\theta^2(1 - \theta)^2$	$\dfrac{1}{4}\theta^2(1 - \theta)^2$	$\dfrac{1}{4}\theta^4$

Similarly, if the fetus (II3) inherits an AB genotype, the probability that it will be affected equals the sum of

   a. $(1) \times (1 - \theta)\theta$ plus
   b. $(2) \times (1 - \theta)^2$ plus
   c. $(3) \times \theta^2$ plus
   d. $(4) \times \theta(1 - \theta)$,

and if the fetus (II3) inherits a BB genotype, the probability that it will be affected equals the sum of

   a. $(1) \times \theta^2$ plus
   b. $(2) \times \theta(1 - \theta)$ plus
   c. $(3) \times (1 - \theta)\theta$ plus
   d. $(4) \times (1 - \theta)^2$

Review of the probabilities that the disease genes in the parents are in coupling with A or B, i.e., probabilities 1–4, reveals that value 1 will be very much greater than any of the others. For example, for values of $\theta = 0.01$ and 0.05, the posterior probability that the disease gene is in coupling with A in both parents equals 0.9998 and 0.9945, respectively. Hence, for the example shown in Figure 5.6, it would be reasonable to proceed on the basis that the linkage phase in the parents is known with certainty. Consequently, if the fetus (II3) inherits an AA genotype, the probability that it will be affected equals $(1 - \theta)^2$, which equals $1 - 2\theta + \theta^2$ and approximates to $1 - 2\theta$. If the fetus inherits an AB (or BA) genotype, the probability that it will be affected equals $2(1 - \theta)\theta$, which equals $2(\theta - \theta^2)$ and approximates to 2θ. Finally, if the fetus inherits a BB genotype, then the probability that it will be affected equals θ^2.

These approximate risk values could have been deduced by simple inspection of the pedigree, which, as the affected sibs show concordance for the marker genotype, indicates that the disease gene in both parents is almost certainly in coupling with marker A. If this is assumed with certainty, then II3 will be affected, given an AA genotype, unless a crossover occurs in either paternal or maternal meiosis. Consequently, the probability that II3 will be affected equals $1 - 2\theta$. If an AB (or BA) genotype is inherited, then II3 will be affected only if a crossover occurs in the parent from whom B is inherited (could be the mother or the father), so that the probability of being affected equals 2θ. Finally, if a BB genotype is inherited, II3 will be affected only if a crossover occurs in both parents, giving a probability of θ^2 of being affected.

Key Point 4

If two or more affected siblings show concordance for closely linked markers, then it is reasonable to assume that the parental linkage phases are known. For a sibling who inherits both, one, or neither of the high-risk linked markers, the probability of being affected equals $1 - 2\theta$, 2θ, and θ^2, respectively.

5.4 X-Linked Recessive Inheritance

Example 6—Phase Unknown

The mother, II2, is known to be a carrier, as she has had two affected sons and an affected brother. Since only one son is available for linkage studies, the phase in the mother is not known with certainty. This situation is similar to that outlined in Example 2, so in this example the calculation will be based on the assumption that III3 has inherited the marker allele different from that in III2.

The probability that the marker gene B in III3 is in coupling with the disease gene equals $\theta(1 - \theta)$ if the disease is in coupling with B in the mother, plus $(1 - \theta)\theta$ if the disease is in coupling with A in the mother. Therefore, the total probability that marker gene B is in coupling with the disease gene in II3 equals $2\theta - 2\theta^2$. If a value of $\theta = 0.05$ is assumed, as is the case for many of the linked markers used for DMD, then the probability that III3 in Figure 5.7 will be affected if he inherits allele B equals 9.5%.

Example 7: Mother's Carrier Status Unknown

II1 represents an isolated case of a genetically lethal X-linked recessive disorder such as DMD. The approach to this problem has been considered at length in Chapter 4. The use of linked markers provides additional information that may modify the likelihood that the mother or sister of this affected boy is a carrier (Fig. 5.8). The calculation proceeds as shown in Table 5.4.

This table shows that the posterior probability that the mother (I2) is a carrier equals

$$\frac{2 - 4\theta + 4\theta^2}{3 - 4\theta + 4\theta^2}$$

which equals 0.644 if $\theta = 0.05$.

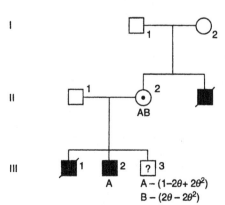

Figure 5.7. X-linked recessive inheritance. Values for the probability that III3 will be affected given different marker genotypes are indicated.

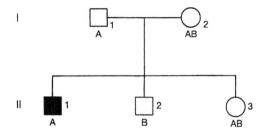

Figure 5.8. II1 represents an isolated case of an X-linked recessive lethal disorder. A and B are allelic markers closely linked to the disease locus.

Now consider the sister, II3, who wishes to know the probability that she is a carrier. For her mother, the probability that she is a carrier with the disease in coupling with A equals

$$\frac{2 - 4\theta + 2\theta^2}{3 - 4\theta + 4\theta^2} \tag{1}$$

which equals approximately 0.642 if $\theta = 0.05$.

Similarly, the probability that I2 is a carrier with the disease in coupling with B equals

$$\frac{2\theta^2}{3 - 4\theta + 4\theta^2} \tag{2}$$

which equals approximately 0.002 if $\theta = 0.05$.

Therefore, the probability that the sister (II3) is a carrier equals $[(1) \times \theta]$ plus $[(2) \times (1 - \theta)]$ since she has inherited allele B from her mother. If $\theta = 0.05$, this gives a value of approximately 1 in 30, a much lower value than the risk of 1 in 4 that would have been derived without linkage information (see Chapter 4).

Example 8: Carrier Test Results Available

Information provided by the results of carrier tests can also be incorporated into these calculations. Consider once again the mother discussed in Example 7 (I2 in

Table 5.4.

Probability	Mother (I2) a Carrier		Mother (I2) Not a Carrier
	Disease in Coupling with A	Disease in Coupling with B	
Prior	2μ	2μ	1
Conditional			
Affected son has A	$(1 - \theta)$	θ	μ
Normal son has B	$(1 - \theta)$	θ	1
Joint	$2\mu(1 - \theta)^2$	$2\mu\theta^2$	μ

Table 5.5.

Probability	Mother a Carrier		Mother not a Carrier
	Disease in Coupling with A	Disease in Coupling with B	
Prior	2μ	2μ	1
Conditional			
CK results	2	2	1
Affected son has inherited A	$1 - \theta$	θ	μ
Unaffected son has inherited B	$1 - \theta$	θ	1
Joint	$4\mu(1 - \theta)^2$	$4\mu\theta^2$	μ

CK, creatine kinase.

Fig. 5.8). If serial creatine kinase estimations give a 2:1 ratio for carrier:noncarrier, then this 2:1 ratio can be included as an additional conditional probability, as in Table 5.5.

This gives a posterior probability of

$$\frac{4 - 8\theta + 8\theta^2}{5 - 8\theta + 8\theta^2}$$

that the mother is a carrier, which equals approximately 0.78 if $\theta = 0.05$. Thus, unfavorable creatine kinase results have increased the probability that the mother is a carrier from 0.64 (Example 7) to 0.78.

5.5 Using Information from Flanking Markers

The use of flanking markers that bridge the disease locus can greatly enhance diagnostic precision, although the ensuing risk calculation can be remarkably difficult (Winter, 1985). Two examples are considered to illustrate the potential value of this approach. In Example 9, both the disease status and the linkage phase in the affected parent of the individual at risk are known. In Example 10, neither the carrier status nor the linkage phase is known. In both of these examples, the possibility that the occurrence of one crossover influences the likelihood that another closely adjacent crossover can occur is ignored. This phenomenon is referred to as *interference*.

Example 9

Information is sought about the probable disease status of III1 (Fig. 5.9), who is at risk of inheriting his mother's late-onset autosomal dominant disorder. It is apparent that the disease allele in the mother (II2) must be in coupling with A1 and B1. Thus, if III1 inherits both A1 and B1 from his mother, there is a high probability that he will also have inherited the disease. In contrast, if III1 inherits both A2 and B2 from his mother, there is an equally high probability that he will not have inherited the

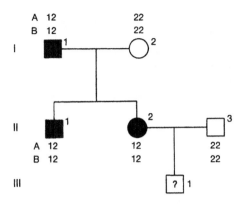

Figure 5.9. A and B represent loci closely linked to and bridging the disease locus. 1 and 2 represent polymorphic alleles at each of these linked loci.

Table 5.6.

Haplotype Inherited from II2		Relative Likelihood of Inheriting Disease Gene	Relative Likelihood of Not Inheriting Disease Gene
A	B		
1	1	$(1 - \theta_A)(1 - \theta_B) = \dfrac{361}{400}$	$\theta_A \theta_B = \dfrac{1}{400}$
1	2	$(1 - \theta_A)(\theta_B) = \dfrac{19}{400}$	$\theta_A(1 - \theta_B) = \dfrac{19}{400}$
2	1	$\theta_A(1 - \theta_B) = \dfrac{19}{400}$	$(1 - \theta_A)\theta_B = \dfrac{19}{400}$
2	2	$\theta_A \theta_B = \dfrac{1}{400}$	$(1 - \theta_A)(1 - \theta_B) = \dfrac{361}{400}$

disease. The precise values of these probabilities are given in Table 5.6. (The values indicated are those obtained if $\theta_A = \theta_B = 0.05$.)

If III1 inherits A1 and B1 from his mother, the odds are 361:1 that he will be affected, i.e., a probability of $361/362 = 0.997$. This is obviously much greater than the value of 0.95 obtained using a single linked marker. If III1 inherits A1 and B2, the odds are 19:19 that he will be affected, i.e., a probability of $19/38 = 0.5$. An identical risk is obtained if III1 inherits A2 and B1. Both of these crossover haplotypes mean that the predictive test is not informative. Inheritance of an A2:B2 haplotype will convey an extremely low risk of 1/362.

Example 10

This example is included to show just how complex the estimation of risks can be when using flanking markers. In Figure 5.10, II1 represents an isolated case of a genetically lethal X-linked recessive disorder such as DMD. It will be remembered from Chapter 4 that in this situation there is a probability of 2/3 that the mother is a carrier, and hence a probability of 1/3 that the sister (II2) is a carrier. Linked bridging markers can be used to modify this risk for the sister. The actual calculation

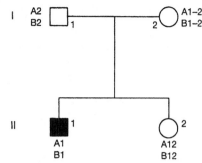

Figure 5.10. II1 represents an isolated
case of Duchenne muscular dystrophy. A and B
are closely linked bridging markers.

from first principles is formidable and is illustrated in Table 5.7. To make the
calculation manageable, it is assumed that $\theta_A = \theta_B$. From Table 5.7, it is possible to
calculate that if the sister inherits the same A1B1 haplotype from her mother as did
her brother, then the probability that she is a carrier is

$$\frac{1-4\theta+8\theta^2-8\theta^3+4\theta^4}{1.5-6\theta+18\theta^2-24\theta^3+12\theta^4} \tag{1}$$

Thus, if $\theta = 0$ the probability for carrier status will be identical to that of the mother,
i.e., 2/3. If $\theta = 0.05$, then equation (1) gives a value of 0.66 for the probability of
being a carrier.

Similarly, it can be shown by an equally difficult calculation that the probability
that II2 is a carrier if she inherits the A2B2 haplotype from her mother is

$$\frac{4\theta^2 - 8\theta^3 + 4\theta^4}{1.5-6\theta+18\theta^2-24\theta^3+12\theta^4} \tag{2}$$

This gives a value of 0 if $\theta = 0$, and of 0.007 if $\theta = 0.05$

In summary, if the daughter inherits the same haplotype as her brother, then the
probability that she is a carrier will be close to 2/3 if θ is small, whereas if she
inherits the different haplotype, then the probability of being a carrier will be very
small and close to 0 if θ is small. If the daughter inherits A1B2 or B1A2, then the
probability of being a carrier will be 1/3, i.e., half of her mother's probability, as
there will be a probability of 0.5 that the crossover will have included or excluded
the disease gene.

Key Point 5

The use of polymorphic markers that flank the disease locus reduces the possibility
of predictive error caused by a single crossover. However, if a single crossover
does occur between the flanking markers, then the predictive test becomes uninfor-
mative.

Table 5.7. Derivation of the Probability That II2 in Figure 5.10 (Example 10) Is a Carrier

Probability	I2 is a Carrier				I2 Is Not a Carrier			
	A1 — Disease — B1	A1 — Disease — B2	A2 — Disease — B1	A2 — Disease — B2	A1 — B1	A2 — B2	A1 — B2	A2 — B1
Prior	μ	μ	μ	μ	$\tfrac{1}{2}$		$\tfrac{1}{2}$	
Conditional	1*				2*			
(1) affected son (II1) with A1B1	$\tfrac{1}{2}(1-\theta)^2$	$\tfrac{1}{2}(1-\theta)\theta$	$\tfrac{1}{2}\theta(1-\theta)$	$\tfrac{1}{2}\theta^2$	$\mu\tfrac{1}{2}(1-2\theta+2\theta^2)$		$\mu\tfrac{1}{2}(2\theta-2\theta^2)$	
	C / NC	C / NC	C / NC	C / NC	C / NC		C / NC	
(2) daughter (II2) Prior	$\tfrac{1}{2}\ /\ \tfrac{1}{2}$	$\tfrac{1}{2}\ /\ \tfrac{1}{2}$	$\tfrac{1}{2}\ /\ \tfrac{1}{2}$	$\tfrac{1}{2}\ /\ \tfrac{1}{2}$	$2\mu\ /\ 1$		$2\mu\ /\ 1$	
Conditional A1B1	$(1-\theta)^2\ /\ \theta^2$	$(1-\theta)\theta\ /\ \theta(1-\theta)$	$(1-\theta)\theta\ /\ \theta(1-\theta)$	$\theta^2\ /\ (1-\theta)^2$	$\tfrac{1}{2}(1-2\theta+2\theta^2)\ /\ \tfrac{1}{2}(2\theta-2\theta^2)$		$\tfrac{1}{2}(1-2\theta+2\theta^2)\ /\ \tfrac{1}{2}(2\theta-2\theta^2)$	
Joint	a / b	c / d	e / f	g / h	i / j		k / l	

Posterior probability for daughter (II2) being a carrier $= \dfrac{(a+c+e+g+i+k)}{(a+b+c+d+e+f+g+h+i+j+k+l)}$

The conditional probabilities 1 and 2 are derived as follows:

1. If the disease is in coupling with A1 and B1 in I2, then the probability of observing II1 will be $\tfrac{1}{2}$ (the probability that II1 inherits A1) $\times (1-\theta)^2$ (the probability that II1 also inherits the disease and B1).

2. If I2 is not a carrier, the probability of observing II1 will be μ (the probability that a mutation has occurred on the X chromosome II1 inherits from I2) $\times \tfrac{1}{2}$ (the probability that II1 inherits A1) $\times [1-2\theta+2\theta^2]$ (the probability that II1 also inherits B1 with either no intervening crossover $(1-\theta)^2$ or as a result of two crossovers $(\theta)^2$).

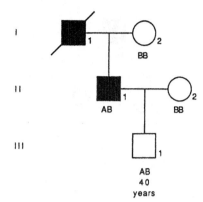

Figure 5.11. III1 is aged 40 years and wishes to know the probability that he has inherited Huntington disease from his father.

Table 5.8.

Probability	III1 Has Inherited Disease	III1 Has Not Inherited Disease
Prior	$1 - \theta$	θ
Conditional		
Age 40 years and unaffected	0.7	1
Joint	$0.7(1 - \theta)$	θ

5.6 Disorders with Late Onset

Many important autosomal dominant disorders show onset at variable age in adult life. For most of these disorders, linked markers are available that can be used to modify risks. Three examples are considered.

Example 11: Disease Phase Known

In Figure 5.11, III1 is aged 40 years and wishes to know the probability that he will develop a disorder such as Huntington's disease, which has affected both his father and his grandfather. The disease in his father II1 must be in coupling with marker A, and III1 has inherited this allele from his father. The calculation proceeds as in Table 5.8.

If $\theta = 0.05$, this gives a posterior probability of 0.93 that III1 has inherited the disease gene from his father, only slightly less than the risk of 95% that would have existed using just information from the linked marker. The conditional probability of 0.7 for III1 being unaffected at age 40 years was obtained from Table 2.9, which indicates that 30% of Huntington's disease heterozygotes show clinical signs of disease by that age.

Example 12: Disease Phase Not Known

In Figure 5.12, II3 wishes to know the probability that he has inherited Huntington's disease from his father I1, who is no longer alive. This individual's marker genotype

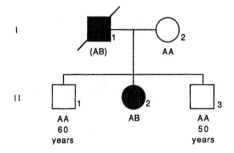

Figure 5.12. II3 is aged 50 years and wishes to know the probability that he has inherited Huntington disease from his father.

Table 5.9.

Probability	Disease in I1 in Coupling with A		Disease in I1 in Coupling with B	
Prior	0.5		0.5	
Conditional				
I11 (AA) is well aged 60 years	$[(1 - \theta) \times 0.25] + \theta$		$(\theta \times 0.25) + (1 - \theta)$	
II2 (AB) is affected	θ		$1 - \theta$	
II3(AA)	Has inherited disease	Has not inherited disease	Has inherited disease	Has not inherited disease
Prior	$1 - \theta$	θ	θ	$1 - \theta$
Conditional				
Well at age 50 years	0.5	1	0.5	1
Joint	a	b	c	d

can be deduced as having been AB by inspection of the pedigree. The risk for II3 is calculated as in Table 5.9, where the value of 0.25 indicates the probability that a 60-year-old heterozygote would be unaffected (Table 2.9).

From this Bayesian table the posterior probability that II3 has inherited the disease, given that he is unaffected at age 50 years and has inherited marker A from his father, equals

$$\frac{a + c}{a + b + c + d}$$

which equals 0.033 (1/30) if $\theta = 0.05$.

Example 13: Disease Phase Not Known

In Figure 5.13, II3 is aged 50 years and wishes to know the likelihood that she has inherited Huntington's disease from her deceased father. Once again, the father's genotype can be deduced by simple inspection of the pedigree. The risk to II3 is calculated as in Table 5.10.

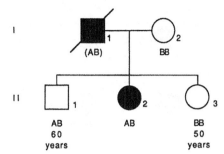

Figure 5.13. II3 is aged 50 years and wishes to know the probability that she has inherited Huntington' disease from her deceased father.

Table 5.10.

Probability	Disease in I1 in Coupling with A		Disease in I1 in Coupling with B	
Prior	0.5		0.5	
Conditional				
I1 (AB) is well aged 60 years	$[(1 - \theta) \times 0.25] + \theta$		$(\theta \times 0.25) + (1 - \theta)$	
II2 (AB) is affected	$1 - \theta$		θ	
II3(BB)	Has Inherited disease	Has Not inherited disease	Has Inherited disease	Has Not inherited Disease
Prior	θ	$1 - \theta$	$1 - \theta$	θ
Conditional				
Well at age 50 years	0.5	1	0.5	1
Joint	a	b	c	d

From this table, the posterior probability that II3 has inherited the disease, given that she is unaffected at age 50 years and has inherited marker B from her father, equals

$$\frac{a + c}{a + b + c + d}$$

which equals 0.101 if $\theta = 0.05$.

In this family the information provided by I1 suggests that the disease in I1 is likely to be in coupling with marker B. However, the information provided by II2 and II3 points toward the disease in I1 being in coupling with marker A, giving an overall risk to II3 of approximately 10% for developing Huntington's disease.

5.7 Parental Genotypes Not Known

It is readily apparent that when counseling for autosomal dominant disorders, it is desirable to have information available from two or preferably three generations. Unfortunately, all too often, information can only be obtained from one generation.

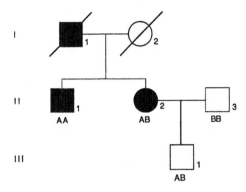

Figure 5.14. Parental genotypes
are not known and cannot be deduced.
Details of the risk calculation for III1 are
given in Table 5.11.

However, this does not mean that linked markers cannot be used for predictive purposes. The following example illustrates how this can be achieved.

Example 14

In Figure 5.14, III1 wishes to know the probability that he has inherited a late-onset disorder from his mother, II2. The maternal grandparents of III1 have both died, and their genotypes for the linked markers cannot be deduced. To simplify matters, III1 is relatively young and has not yet lived through any significant risk period, so he does not contribute any information regarding the likely linkage phase in his mother.

The calculation is approached by constructing Table 5.11, which is based on all possible genotypes for I1 and I2. In assigning the prior probabilities for each of these possible matings, it has been assumed that only two alleles (A and B) exist at the marker locus and that each of these has an equal gene frequency. Thus, the prior probability ratios for matings AA × AA, AA × AB, and AB × AB will be 1:2:4, as heterozygotes will be twice as common as homozygotes. The conditional probabilities are determined by establishing, for example in mating 4, the probability that I1 will inherit the specified paternal marker A $(1/2)$, be affected $(1 - \theta)$, and also inherit the maternal marker A$(1/2)$, giving a total of $1/2(1 - \theta)1/2$.

From Table 5.11, the probability that the disease is in coupling with marker A in II2 can be determined by summating a, d, and f and dividing this by the sum of a to g inclusive. If $\theta = 0.05$, a value of 0.87 is obtained. Conversely, the probability that the disease is in coupling with marker B in II2 equals 0.13. Thus, the probability that III1 has inherited the disease equals $(0.87 \times 0.95) + (0.13 \times 0.05)$, which equals approximately 0.83.

Key Point 6

When the relevant parental marker genotypes are unknown and cannot be deduced, it is still possible to determine offspring risks by drawing up a Bayesian table that includes a column for each possible combination of parental disease–marker haplotypes.

Table 5.11. Derivation of the Probability That the Disease in II2 (Fig 5.14 (Example 14) Is Coupled with Either Marker A or Marker B

	1		2		3		4			5		
Parental genotype (I1 and I2)	AA	AB	AB	AA	AB	AA	AB	AB		AB	AB	
			HC		HC		HC			HC		
Probability												
Prior (= relative frequency of mating)	2		1		1		2			2		
Conditional III AA and affected	$\frac{1}{2} \times \frac{1}{2}$		$\frac{1}{2}(1-\theta)$		$\frac{1}{2}\theta$		$\frac{1}{2}(1-\theta)\frac{1}{2}$			$\frac{1}{2}(\theta)\frac{1}{2}$		
							Pat A Mat B	Pat B Mat A		Pat A Mat B	Pat B Mat A	
II2 AB and affected	$\frac{1}{2} \times \frac{1}{2}$		$\frac{1}{2}\theta$		$\frac{1}{2}(1-\theta)$		$\frac{1}{2}(1-\theta)\frac{1}{2}$	$\frac{1}{2}\theta\frac{1}{2}$		$\frac{1}{2}\theta\frac{1}{2}$	$\frac{1}{2}(1-\theta)\frac{1}{2}$	
Joint	a		b		c		d	e		f	g	
HC in II2 coupled with	A		B		B		A	B		A	B	

5.8 Linkage Disequilibrium

The term *linkage disequilibrium* relates to the situation in which particular alleles at linked loci occur together on the same chromosome more or less frequently than would be expected by chance. If two linked loci, A and B, each have two alleles, A1 A2 and B1 B2, with allele frequencies of pl(A1), p2(A2), q1(B1), and q2(B2), then if equilibrium exists, the following haplotype frequencies should be observed:

Haplotype	A1B1	A1B2	A2B1	A2B2
Frequency	plq1	plq2	p2q1	p2q2

Statistically significant deviation from these frequencies would provide evidence for linkage disequilibrium. Linkage disequilibrium can be viewed as a "snapshot" phenomenon observed during the evolution of a population. When it has been demonstrated between a disease allele and a closely linked DNA polymorphism, it strongly suggests that the disease mutation has arisen relatively recently in a single common ancestor or that the DNA marker is located on a highly "mutable" chromosome. Whatever the explanation, the demonstration of strong linkage disequilibrium between a disease allele and an identifiable closely adjacent polymorphic DNA marker can be used to modify risks in the interval before the disease allele itself has been identified.

This is illustrated using the example of cystic fibrosis. Shortly before the gene was isolated, it was demonstrated in European and North American populations that cystic fibrosis mutations showed very strong linkage disequilibrium with several very tightly linked DNA markers including those identified using the XV-2c and KM-19 probes (Beaudet et al., 1989). In the North American population, the haplotype consisting of the XV-2c allele (1) and the KM-19 allele (2) was found on 218 out of 252 ($= 86.5\%$) cystic fibrosis chromosomes compared with only 35 out of 250 ($= 14\%$) non–cystic fibrosis chromosomes. The following example illustrates how this information was used in risk calculation.

Example 15

The upper half of Figure 5.15 shows the haplotypes for the XV-2c and KM-19 probes in two siblings with cystic fibrosis, their parents, their unaffected sister, and her healthy unrelated spouse. Since a crossover between the tightly linked marker and disease loci is highly improbable, it is apparent that in both parents the cystic fibrosis gene is almost certainly in coupling with a high-risk XV-2c(1)/KM-19(2) haplotype, as indicated in the lower half of Figure 5.15. It is also apparent that the healthy sister has therefore inherited one cystic fibrosis allele and is thus a carrier.

The healthy sister, II3, and her equally healthy and unrelated spouse, II4, wish to know the probability that their first child will have cystic fibrosis. For this to be determined, it is necessary to know the probability that II4 is a carrier. This is calculated as follows, remembering that the XV-2c(1)/KM-19(2) haplotype is found on 86.5% of cystic fibrosis chromosomes and 14% of non–cystic fibrosis chromosomes and assuming, for the sake of convenience, that the cystic fibrosis gene has a frequency of 1 in 50.

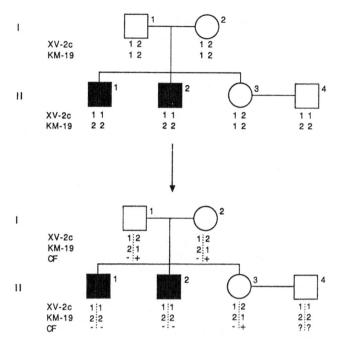

Figure 5.15. The two affected boys have cystic fibrosis. Haplotypes obtained using the XV-2c and KM-19 probes are indicated. + is the normal allele; − is the cystic fibrosis allele.

Consider 1000 chromosomes in the general population. Twenty of these carry a cystic fibrosis mutation, of which $20 \times 0.865 (= 17.3)$ have the high-risk haplotype. The remaining 980 chromosomes do not carry a cystic fibrosis mutation. Of these, $980 \times 0.14 (= 137.2)$ carry the high-risk haplotype. Thus, for any chromosome with this XV-2c(1)/KM-19(2) haplotype there is a probability of $17.3/(17.3 + 137.2)$ that it also carries the cystic fibrosis gene. This equals 0.112 or approximately 1 in 9.

Hence, for the healthy sister's spouse, II4, there is a probability of $1/9 \times 1/9$ that he is homozygous affected, $8/9 \times 8/9$ that he is homozygous unaffected, and $2 \times 1/9 \times 8/9$ that he is heterozygous. The probabilities are as follows:

homozygous affected—1/81
heterozygous (carrier)—16/81
homozygous unaffected—64/81

Since II4 is known to be in good health, it can safely be assumed that he does not have cystic fibrosis, so the overall probability that he is a carrier equals $16/(16 + 64)$, which equals 0.2 or 1/5.

Returning to Figure 5.15, it is now possible to inform the healthy sister and her spouse that there is a probability of approximately 1 in 20 (i.e., $1 \times 1/5 \times 1/4$) that their first baby will be affected with cystic fibrosis. This will rise to 1/10 if the fetus is found to have inherited its mother's cystic fibrosis chromosome. Without this information, provided by knowledge of the linkage disequilibrium, the healthy sister and her spouse would have been informed of a much lower risk ($2/3 \times 1/25 \times 1/4 = 1/150$) of having an affected child.

In practice, it is unusual for knowledge of linkage disequilibrium to be used for risk calculation, as most of the disease-causing genes for which it has been demonstrated have been isolated. Occasionally, it can still be of value. For example, the healthy brother of a deceased sibling with cystic fibrosis may want to know his carrier status. If mutation detection in both the healthy brother and his parents proves unhelpful, then knowledge of linkage disequilibrium can be used to show if the brother has inherited a high-risk haplotype from one of his parents.

5.9 Linkage Heterogeneity

Several apparently homogeneous genetic disorders show nonallelic heterogeneity. Important examples include tuberous sclerosis and adult polycystic kidney disease. If nonallelic heterogeneity has been established for a particular disorder, this should be taken into account when using linked markers for risk calculation.

A very small pedigree may not provide any information about the likelihood that the disease in that particular family is linked with the marker locus being studied. This would apply to the family shown in Figure 5.3 (Example 2). If it has been established from extensive research that the disease segregates with the marker locus in, say, 90% of families, then this information can be taken into account in the risk calculation in the following way. For II2 in Figure 5.3, the probability that she will be affected, given that she has inherited marker A from her father, will be 0.9 (= the proportion of families showing linkage with the marker locus) $\times$ $(1 - 2\theta + 2\theta^2)$ (= the probability that she will be affected if the disease in the family is linked with the marker locus), plus 0.1 (= the proportion of families not showing linkage with the marker locus) $\times$ 0.5 (the pedigree risk to II2 given autosomal dominant inheritance with complete penetrance).

Example 16

A larger pedigree can provide information about the probability that the disease is cosegregating with the marker locus. Figure 5.16 shows an X-linked recessive pedigree with A and B representing allelic polymorphic markers at a locus closely

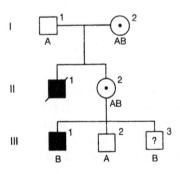

Figure 5.16. The X-linked recessive disorder segregating in this family shows locus heterogeneity. Calculation of the risk for III3 must therefore take into account the possibility that the marker locus is not linked with the disease locus.

Table 5.12.

Probability	Disease Focus Linked with Marker Focus (Therefore, Disease in II2 Is in Coupling with B)	Disease Focus Not Linked with Marker Focus
Prior	0.8	0.2
Conditional		
III1 has inherited B and is affected	$1 - \theta$	0.5
III2 has inherited A and is not affected	$1 - \theta$	0.5
Joint	$0.8(1 - \theta)^2$	0.05

linked to the disease locus in 80% of families but not showing linkage ($\theta = 0.5$) in the remaining 20%. In this pedigree II2 is an obligatory carrier, and if the disease is linked to the marker locus, then in II2 the disease gene must be in coupling with marker B, since both the disease and marker B have been inherited on the X chromosome from I2. The information provided by III1 and III2 is consistent with the disease gene in II2 being in coupling with marker B, and therefore increases the probability that the disease in the family is cosegregating with the marker locus. The probability that III3 will be affected, given that he inherits marker B, is calculated by first determining the new probability that the disease is cosegregating with the marker locus (Table 5.12) and then proceeding as in the previous paragraph.

The posterior probability that the disease is cosegregating with the marker locus equals

$$\frac{0.8(1 - \theta)^2}{0.8(1 - \theta)^2 + 0.05}$$

which approximates to 0.935 if $\theta = 0.05$. Therefore, the probability that III3 will be affected equals [$0.935 \times (1 - \theta)$] plus [$0.065 \times 0.5$], giving an overall risk of approximately 0.92, only slightly less than the risk of 0.95 that would apply if the disorder were known to be genetically homogeneous.

This example demonstrates how nonallelic genetic heterogeneity can be catered for in relatively simple pedigrees. In more complex situations, use of a computer program is essential. This has been discussed in relation to X-linked agammaglobulinemia by Lau et al. (1988).

Key Point 7

Locus heterogeneity should be taken into account when calculating risks using linked markers. Information from a large pedigree will often indicate at which locus the disease is most likely to be segregating. This information should be included in the overall calculation. In a small pedigree, risks can be calculated using the prior probabilities of linkage to each locus obtained from population studies.

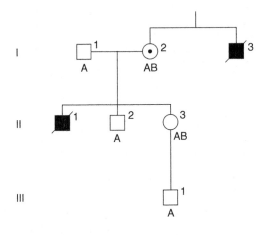

Figure 5.17. I3 and II1 were both affected with Duchenne muscular dystrophy. A and B represent allelic intragenic polymorphisms. The calculation of the probability that II3 is a carrier is shown in Table 5.13.

5.10 Case Scenario

Figure 5.17 shows the pedigree of a family in which two boys, I3 and II1, have died with a diagnosis of DMD, which is caused by mutations in the dystrophin gene. No dystrophin mutation has been identified in the obligate carrier I2. Her daughter, II3, wishes to know the probability that she is a carrier. The results of testing with an informative intragenic polymorphic marker are indicated. This marker is located in the middle of the dystrophin gene, with an estimated average recombination fraction between the marker and disease mutations of 0.05. Creatine phosphokinase testing in II3 yields conditional odds of 2:1 in favor of being a carrier.

Using the Bayesian calculation shown in Table 5.13, it can be shown that the probability that II3 is a carrier equals approximately 0.95. This high risk is derived mainly from the observation that II3 and her unaffected brother, II2, have inherited

Table 5.13   (see Case Scenario and Fig. 5.17).

| Probability | I2 Is a Carrier | | | |
	Disease Linked with A		Disease Linked with B	
Prior	$\frac{1}{2}$		$\frac{1}{2}$	
Conditional				
II2 is not affected	θ		$1-\theta$	
II3 inherits B from I2	C	NC	C	NC
	θ	$1-\theta$	$1-\theta$	θ
II1 is not affected	$1-\theta$	1	$1-\theta$	1
CPK result in II3	2	1	2	1
	$\theta^2(1-\theta)$	$\frac{1}{2}\theta(1-\theta)$	$1-(\theta)^3$	$\frac{1}{2}\theta(1-\theta)$

Posterior probability that II3 is a carrier equals $[\theta^2(1-\theta)+(1-\theta)^3]/[\theta^2(1-\theta)+(1-\theta)^3+\frac{1}{2}\theta(1-\theta)+\frac{1}{2}\theta(1-\theta)]$, which reduces to $(1-2\theta+2\theta^2)/(1-\theta+2\theta^2)=0.948$ if $\theta=0.05$.

different dystrophin genes from their mother. Using information provided only by the linked marker, the probability that II3 is a carrier would equal approximately 0.91. Based on the pedigree and the creatine kinase results alone, the probability that II3 is a carrier would equal 0.5.

Further Reading

Bridge, P.J. (1997). *The calculation of genetic risks. Worked examples in DNA diagnostics*, 2nd ed. Johns Hopkins University Press, Baltimore.

Kadasi, L. (1989). Estimating the error rate in DNA diagnosis with linked markers. *Human Heredity*, **39**, 67–74.

Ott, J. (1999). *Analysis of human genetic linkage*. Johns Hopkins University Press, Baltimore.

Strachan, T. and Read, A.P. (2004). *Human molecular genetics 3*. Garland Science, New York.

6

Germline Mosaicism

The issue of germline mosaicism has generated a great deal of uncertainty in the provision of genetic risks over the past 10–15 years. Previously, this was not perceived to be a major concern. Rare reports of siblings with conditions such as campomelic dysplasia, severe osteogenesis imperfecta, and pseudoachondroplasia, born to unaffected parents, were attributed to autosomal recessive inheritance or other mechanisms such as independent mutations. There was little appreciation that germline mosaicism is a common occurrence until molecular analysis began to reveal that in DMD the recurrence risk for an apparently de novo mutation can be as high as 10%. Subsequent studies confirmed that germline mosaicism is seen in many conditions and should always be considered when estimating genetic risks.

Unfortunately, despite extensive study, no simple mathematical model has emerged that allows the possibility of germline mosaicism to be catered for in straightforward Mendelian or Bayesian calculations. In the previous edition of this book, coverage of this important subject was dispersed throughout three chapters, with an extended appendix in which several complex mathematical approaches were presented. These were not particularly easy to understand. In this edition, this subject is considered in this chapter, with less erudite but more practical guidelines as to how the problems generated by germline mosaicism can be approached.

6.1 What Is Germline Mosaicism?

Traditionally, it was assumed that new mutations arise in meiosis, so that unaffected parents of a newly affected child could in theory be counseled on the basis of a negligible recurrence risk in a future pregnancy. In reality, it is now known that this is incorrect and that many "new" mutations arise in a mitotic division, so that a variable and unpredictable proportion of cells in the relevant parent will harbor the pathogenic mutation. This presence of two cell lines with different genetic constitutions in an individual, who is derived from a single zygote, is referred to as *mosaicism*. If the mutation occurs in an early somatic division in the developing embryo, so that it is present in both somatic and gonadal cells, then this is referred to as *gonosomal mosaicism*. If the mutation arises in a mitotic division in one of the parental gonads, this is referred to as *gonadal* or *germline mosaicism*. Both gonosomal and germline mosaicism have important implications for genetic counseling.

6.2 A Simplified Model of Gametogenesis

In devising a comprehensible approach to the derivation of risks for germline mosaicism, it is assumed that gametogenesis involves a synchronous symmetrical process of cell division commencing with a single germline progenitor cell (Fig 6.1) (Edwards, 1989; Hartl, 1971). This process differs radically in males and females (Crow, 2000). In the female, it has been estimated that there are a total of 22 mitotic divisions followed by the single replication that precedes meiosis prior to the birth of a female infant. Thereafter the gametes are quiescent and undergo no further cell divisions. In the male, approximately 30 cell divisions occur prior to the onset of puberty, followed by a single stem cell division every 16 days, i.e., approximately 23 per year. Four further mitotic replications and a single meiotic DNA replication

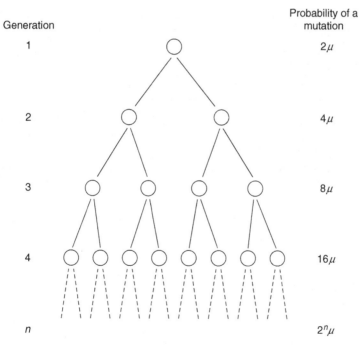

Figure 6.1. Simplified model of gametogenesis showing the probability of mutation in each generation for an autosomal gene. See Tables 6.2 and 6.3.

Table 6.1. Estimated Number of Cell Divisions
(DNA Replications) Undergone by a Mature
Haploid Gamete

Gender	Age (years)	Number of Divisions
Female	All ages	23
Male	15	30–35
	20	150
	25	265
	30	380
	35	495
	40	610
	45	725
	50	840

occur to yield mature gametes. This means that mature sperm produced by older males have gone through large numbers of cell divisions (Table 6.1), each of which provides an opportunity for mutation as a result of a DNA copy error and/or failure of DNA repair. The paternal age effect, as demonstrated by fathers of children with new autosomal dominant mutations being older than average, is probably a direct consequence of this increasing number of mitotic divisions in the germline of older males.

Recurrence Risk After a Single Affected Child

Assume that unaffected parents have had one affected child. If it is accepted that the process of cell division in gamete formation is indeed dichotomous, synchronous, and symmetrical, and that the mutation rate is constant throughout, then it can be shown that if a mutation has occurred (i.e., unaffected parents have had an affected child), there is an equal chance that it has arisen in each of the n generations involved in the production of the gamete (Table 6.2). This conclusion assumes that the probability of ascertainment will be a function of the number of mitoses in each generation (i.e., opportunities for mutation to occur) multiplied by the proportion of

Table 6.2. Determination of the Relative Probability of Ascertainment for a Mutation in Each Generation After a Single Affected Child

	Generation				
	1	2	3	4	n
Probability of a mutation (a)	2μ	4μ	8μ	16μ	$2^n\mu$
Proportion of mutant gametes (b)	$\frac{1}{2}$	$\frac{1}{4}$	$\frac{1}{8}$	$\frac{1}{16}$	$\left(\frac{1}{2}\right)^n$
Probability of ascertaining a mutant gamete (a × b)	μ	μ	μ	μ	μ
Relative probability of ascertainment	1	1	1	1	1

gametes affected if a mutation does occur. This product is equal for each generation. For example, the probability that the single cell in generation 1 will harbor a mutation is 2μ (each cell has two chromosomes—hence two opportunities for a mutation to occur), and if a mutation has occurred, then all of the cells will carry the mutation until meiosis, after which it will be present in half of the gametes ($2\mu \times 1/2 = \mu$ in Table 6.2). Similarly, if the mutation occurs in the next generation, then there will be four chromosomes in which it can take place (probability therefore equals 4μ), but in this instance it will be present in only one-quarter of the gametes ($4\mu \times 1/4 = \mu$ in Table 6.2), and so on. Essentially, this means that there is an equal chance that the mutation has occurred in each generation.

By extending this theme, the recurrence risk can be calculated as follows. If the mutation has occurred in the first generation, the proportion of affected gametes (i.e., the recurrence risk) equals 1/2 (all diploid gametes will carry the mutation, but mature gametes are haploid—thus, only half will possess the mutation). Thus, the recurrence risk generated by this possibility equals $1/n \times 1/2$. For mutations occurring in the next generation, the recurrence risk will equal $1/n \times 1/4$, and so on. The overall recurrence risk therefore equals

$$(1/n \times 1/2) + (1/n \times 1/4) + (1/n \times 1/8) + (1/n \times 1/16) + \cdots (1/n \times (1/2^n))$$
$$= 1/n(1/2 + 1/4 + 1/8 + 1/16 + \cdots 1/2^n)$$

which conveniently reduces to $1/n$.

If the number of generations is 23, as in the female, the recurrence risk will equal approximately 4%–5% (1/23). For a young male aged 15 years, the recurrence risk will be approximately 3% (1/30). For an older male aged 40 years, the recurrence risk will be 0.16% (1/610).

Recurrence Risk After Two or Three Affected Children

If unaffected parents have had two affected children, then it becomes more likely that the mutation has occurred in an early mitotic division (Table 6.3). Specifically, the probability that it has occurred in the first generation is 1 in 2, in the second

Table 6.3. Determination of the Relative Probability of Ascertainment for a Mutation in Each Generation After Two Affected Children

	Generation				
	1	2	3	4	n
Probability of a mutation (a)	2μ	4μ	8μ	16μ	$2^n\mu$
Proportion of gametes affected (b)	1/2	1/4	1/8	1/16	$1/2^n$
Probability of ascertaining two mutant gametes ($a \times b^2$)	$\mu/2$	$\mu/4$	$\mu/8$	$\mu/16$	$\mu/2^n$
Relative probability of ascertainment	1/2	1/4	1/8	1/16	$1/2^n$

generation 1 in 4, in the third generation 1 in 8, and so on. Thus, the recurrence risk for the next pregnancy equals

$$(1/2 \times 1/2) + (1/4 \times 1/4) + (1/8 \times 1/8) + \cdots (1/2^n \times 1/2^n)$$

which reduces to 1/3.

In the same way, it can be shown that after three affected children the recurrence risk equals $3/7 = 0.429$. These figures have been derived much more elegantly and rigorously by Hartl (1971) and by Edwards (1989). It is hoped that the somewhat pedestrian explanation provided here will enable the reader to understand the basic principles involved and appreciate the rationale behind adopting this approach.

6.3 Applying This Simple Model

In theory, the possibility of germline mosaicism should be taken into consideration every time the parents of a child with an apparently de novo autosomal dominant or X-linked mutation are being counseled. In practice, it has emerged that this appears to be much more important for some disorders, notably DMD and osteogenesis imperfecta type II, than for others, such as achondroplasia and Apert syndrome (Table 6.4).

In DMD it has been shown that the empiric risk to the brother of an affected male with a de novo deletion is approximately 1 in 14 (7%), or 1 in 7 (14%) if the brother inherits the same dystrophin gene (as determined by DNA marker analysis) as his affected sibling. Similarly, for a sister inheriting the same dystrophin gene, there is a probability of 1 in 7 that she will be a carrier (Bakker et al., 1989). Van Essen et al. (1992), in reporting the results of a large multicenter study, concluded that the empiric recurrence risk is even greater. They showed that among the siblings of isolated cases with a new mutation, transmission of the at-risk dystrophin haplotype also resulted in transmission of the DMD mutation in 20% of cases. In familial retinoblastoma it has long been recognized that there is a small but significant recurrence risk of around 5% to the sibling of a de novo bilaterally

Table 6.4. Examples of Disorders in Which Germline Mosaicism Has Been Identified

Disorder	Estimated Recurrence Risk	Reference
Achondroplasia	0.2%	Mettler and Fraser (2000)
Apert syndrome	<1%	Moloney et al. (1996)
Duchenne muscular dystrophy	7%–10%	Bakker et al. (1989)
		Van Essen et al. (1992)
Facioscapulohumeral muscular dystrophy	≈10%	Kohler et al. (1996)
		Van der Maarel and Frants (2005)
Marfan syndrome	<1%	Rantamäki et al. (1999)
Osteogenesis imperfecta type II (lethal type)	6%	Byers et al. (1988)
		Cohn et al. (1990)
Retinoblastoma	5%	Sippel et al. (1998)
Tuberous sclerosis	2%–3%	Rose et al. (1999)

affected case. In the past, this was attributed to nonpenetrance in one of the parents or to low-penetrance alleles (p. 19), but recent studies have revealed that parental somatic or gonosomal mosaicism is an equally plausible explanation (Sippel et al., 1998). In this context the point has already been made that somatic mosaicism is one of several possible explanations for apparent reduced penetrance (p. 19).

In contrast to DMD and retinoblastoma, parental germline mosaicism for many other disorders, such as achondroplasia and Apert syndrome, is very uncommon, as indicated by the dearth of reports of affected siblings born to unaffected parents (Table 6.4). This is supported by the empiric observation of only one recurrence among 443 siblings (0.2%) in a large Canadian study of achondroplasia (Mettler and Fraser, 2000). This figure is comparable to the recurrence risk expected for a disorder associated with a significantly advanced paternal age effect.

Thus, for practical purposes, when considering germline mosaicism, disorders can be broken down into two groups—those with a significant recurrence risk, consistent with an early mitotic mutation in one of the parents, and those with a very low risk, consistent with a meiotic or late mitotic mutation often in association with a markedly advanced paternal age effect. This distinction is probably a reflection of different types of mutation, with the high-risk category involving more complex mutational mechanisms such as deletions (e.g., DMD) and contractions (e.g., facioscapulohumeral muscular dystrophy), whereas paternal age-related point mutations predominate in the low-risk group. However, it would be wrong to accept this as an absolute distinction, as point mutations have been observed in female germline mosaicism for DMD.

6.4 Risk Estimates for Use in Counseling

Given that knowledge of the processes underlying mutagenesis and germline mosaicism is still imperfect, a strong case can be made for resorting to empiric risks if these are available. Estimates for commonly encountered conditions are given in Table 6.4. It is important to emphasize that these figures should be used only after the parents have undergone careful evaluation and examination to ensure that neither of them shows any evidence of somatic mosaicism. If no empiric data are available and it is known that the relevant disorder is caused by a wide spectrum of mutational mechanisms in a large gene, then the index of suspicion for germline mosaicism should be high and it would be wise to err on the side of caution when counseling. Alternatively, if the father is older than average and the relevant disorder is usually caused by a point mutation, then the likelihood of a significant recurrence risk due to germline mosaicism is low.

If it can be established by molecular analysis that the mutation has been inherited from a specific parent, then a reasonable approach to arriving at an estimate of the recurrence risk (RR) involves the use of the simple formula $RR = 1/n$, where n equals the number of cell divisions involved in gametogenesis (Table 6.1). Thus, if the mutation has arisen in the mother, $n = 23$ and the recurrence risk equals approximately 4%–5%. In theory, these figures can be reduced further by the existence of unaffected siblings, particularly if they can be shown to have inherited

Table 6.5. Recurrence Risks for Germline Mosaicism with One Affected Child and a Variable Number of Untyped Unaffected Children and Typed Unaffected Children with the At-Risk Chromosome

		No. of Typed Unaffected Children with the At-Risk Chromosome				
		0	1	2	3	4
No. of untyped	0	0.048	0.018	0.013	0.010	0.008
unaffected children	1	0.033	0.015	0.012	0.009	0.008
	2	0.025	0.013	0.010	0.008	0.007
	3	0.019	0.012	0.009	0.008	0.007
	4	0.016	0.011	0.009	0.007	0.006

Source: From van der Meulen et al. (1995) with permission from the BMJ Publishing Group.

the same at-risk chromosome as the affected child. Van der Meulen et al. (1995) calculated recurrence risks for different sibship structures, assuming that $n = 20$, to take into account the results of DNA studies. These risks are reproduced as Tables 6.5 to 6.8. Inspection of Table 6.5 indicates that the maximum recurrence risk after the birth of one affected child equals 0.048 (4.8%) and is reduced to 0.010 (1%) by the presence of three unaffected siblings with the same at-risk chromosome, or to 0.019 (1.9%) by the presence of three untyped unaffected siblings. After two affected children the maximum recurrence risk is 1 in 3, as derived above, and once again, this is reduced by the existence of unaffected children in the sibship (Table 6.6). If the mutation has been transmitted in the sperm of an older father, then the recurrence risk will be much lower (e.g., $1/610 = 0.16\%$ for a 40-year-old father). If the parental origin of the mutation is not known, an estimate of the recurrence risk can be made by taking the average of the figures derived for both parents.

Finally, it is worth noting that if a pathogenic mutation has been identified in the proband, then it may be possible to obtain an indication of the recurrence risk by arranging for mutation analysis of the father's sperm. The recurrence risk will

Table 6.6. Recurrence Risks for Germline Mosaicism with Two Affected Children and a Variable Number of Untyped Unaffected Children and Typed Unaffected Children with the At-Risk Chromosome

		No. of Typed Unaffected Children with the At-Risk Chromosome				
		0	1	2	3	4
No. of untyped	0	0.333	0.143	0.120	0.100	0.084
unaffected children	1	0.286	0.133	0.111	0.093	0.079
	2	0.240	0.124	0.103	0.087	0.074
	3	0.200	0.115	0.096	0.081	0.069
	4	0.168	0.107	0.089	0.075	0.065

Source: From van der Meulen et al. (1995) with permission from the BMJ Publishing Group.

Table 6.7. Recurrence Risks for Germline Mosaicism with Three Affected Children and a Variable Number of Untyped Unaffected Children and Typed Unaffected Children with the At-Risk Chromosome

		No. of Typed Unaffected Children with the At-Risk Chromosome				
		0	1	2	3	4
No. of untyped	0	0.429	0.200	0.183	0.164	0.145
unaffected children	1	0.400	0.194	0.175	0.156	0.138
	2	0.366	0.187	0.168	0.149	0.131
	3	0.328	0.179	0.160	0.141	0.124
	4	0.290	0.172	0.153	0.134	0.118

Source: From van der Meulen et al. (1995) with permission from the BMJ Publishing Group.

Key Point

It is probable that many pathogenic inherited mutations arise in an early developmental mitotic division rather than in meiosis. Thus, the possibility of germline mosaicism must be considered when counseling the parents of a child who presents as the first affected case in the family.

A suggested strategy is as follows:
1. The parents should be carefully assessed to determine if either shows clinical evidence of somatic mosaicism.
2. If a mutation can be identified in the affected child, mutation analysis should be carried out in blood in both parents and ideally also in the father's sperm.
3. If the mutation is not identified in either parent, the literature should be consulted to establish if there are empiric risk data or if there is information about the spectrum of mutations associated with the relevant disorder.
4. If no empiric risk data exist, reference can be made to theoretical risks (Tables 6.5 to 6.8) to obtain an estimate of the recurrence risk. This applies particularly if the parents are young and the disease gene is large, with a broad mutational spectrum. If the father is older than average and the disorder is usually caused by point mutations, then it is reasonable to offer a lower risk.
5. If the pathogenic mutation has been identified, it is always prudent to offer the option of prenatal diagnosis if this is justified by the severity of the condition.

---

equal the proportion of sperm found to harbor the mutation. In practice, however, this facility is rarely available.

6.5 Case Scenario 1

Figure 6.2 shows the pedigree of a family in which III1 presents as an isolated case of DMD. By the time the diagnosis has been made, his parents have a second son,

Table 6.8. Recurrence Risks for Germline Mosaicism with Four Affected Children and a Variable Number of Untyped Unaffected Children and Typed Unaffected Children with the At-Risk Chromosome

		No. of Typed Unaffected Children with the At-Risk Chromosome				
Recurrence Risk		0	1	2	3	4
No of untyped	0	0.467	0.226	0.216	0.203	0.188
unaffected children	1	0.452	0.222	0.211	0.197	0.181
	2	0.431	0.218	0.206	0.191	0.175
	3	0.406	0.214	0.200	0.185	0.168
	4	0.375	0.209	0.195	0.178	0.161

Source: From van der Meulen et al. (1995) with permission from the BMJ Publishing Group.

III2, who, fortunately, is found not to be affected on the basis of creatine kinase assay. Creatine kinase assay undertaken on the mother, II2, is also normal.

Molecular analysis is carried out on the affected boy and subsequently on other family members, as shown in Figure 6.2. No deletion is identified in the dystrophin gene in III1. The results of linkage analysis using two markers, A and B, at opposite ends of the dystrophin gene with alleles A1, A2, B1, and B2 are as indicated. The recombination fraction (θ) between the two markers is 0.1 (i.e., 1 in 10).

The parents of the affected boy now wish to know the probability that a future son will be affected. Inspection of the pedigree indicates that the brothers, III1 and III2, share the same dystrophin haplotype, which has been inherited from their maternal grandfather. This means that the only way their mother could be a carrier is if a double crossover occurred in the dystrophin gene in the formation of the ovum that led to the conception of one of the brothers. Statistically, the chance of a double crossover is 1 in 100 (0.1^2). Taking this observation into account, together with the mother's low level of creatine kinase, it becomes reasonable to conclude

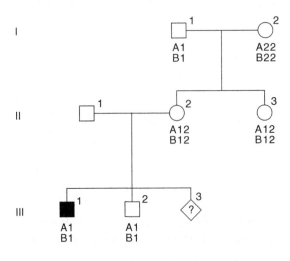

Figure 6.2. III1 presents as an isolated case of Duchenne muscular dystrophy. See Case Scenario 1.

that it is extremely unlikely that the mother is a carrier. This means that the mother's sister, II3, who obviously has inherited the same paternally derived A1B1 dystrophin haplotype, can be reassured that it is equally unlikely that she is a carrier.

Although it is extremely unlikely that the boys' mother is a carrier, it is certainly possible that she is an example of germline mosaicism. Based on the empirically derived recurrence risks of 7%–10% derived by Bakker et al. (1989) and van Essen et al. (1992), which double to 14%–20% for a shared dystrophin haplotype, the probability that III3 will be affected if a male is 14%–20% if he inherits A1B1, less than 1% if he inherits A2B2, and 7%–10% if he inherits A1B2 or A2B1 (indicating that a crossover has occurred).

This case scenario illustrates how a combination of deletion and linkage analysis can be used to predict risk and carrier status in an extended family. The issue of germline mosaicism becomes relevant when the origin of the new mutation has been identified. In this family, the sharing of the haplotype by the affected and unaffected brothers indicated that the mutation must have arisen at some point during gametogenesis in their mother.

6.6 Case Scenario 2

Figure 6.3 shows a family tree that is essentially identical to that shown in Figure 6.2, with the crucial distinction that the younger brother, III2, is found to be affected. As in the previous scenario, no dystrophin deletion is identified. Linkage analysis indicates that both of the affected boys have inherited their maternal grandfather's dystrophin haplotype. On examination, this individual is found to be totally unaffected.

Now there are three possibilities for the origin of the mutation:

1. There was a new meiotic mutation in the germline of I1 resulting in his daughter, II2, being a carrier.

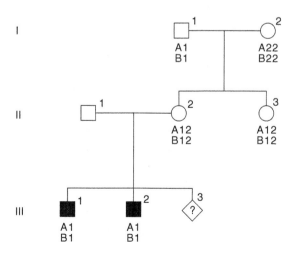

Figure 6.3. Both III1 and III2 are affected with Duchenne muscular dystrophy. See Case Scenario 2.

2. The grandfather, I1, is a germline mosaic.
3. The boys' mother, II2, is a germline mosaic.

(Note that the dystrophin haplotypes make it very unlikely that the mutation was inherited from the maternal grandmother, I2, so that her sisters and their female descendants can be strongly reassured that they are at very low risk for being carriers.)

Unfortunately, there is no validated mathematical model that enables precise prior probabilities to be assigned to each of these three possibilities, so that the use of Bayesian methods to determine overall risks in this situation is problematic (see Appendix A2 in the previous edition of this book). Creatine kinase estimation in II2 might shed light on her carrier status. However, for practical purposes, it makes little difference when counseling II2 whether she is a carrier or a germline mosaic. Either way the recurrence risk for III3 is high, i.e., 1/2 if II2 is a carrier or 1/3 if she is a germline mosaic (Table 6.6). If III3 inherits the A1B1 dystrophin haplotype, these risks are doubled to become 1 or 2/3. These risks are for being affected, if male, or for being a carrier, if female. Determining a carrier risk for the sister of II2, i.e., II3, is much more difficult. Male germline mosaicism for dystrophin point mutations has been reported, but rarely, and its overall contribution to the origin of mutations is unknown. If I1 was relatively young when his daughter, II2, was conceived, then it would be wise to be cautious and counsel on the basis of a low (3%–5%) but far from negligible risk. If I1 was older than average when II2 was conceived, this would point to a lower risk for the carrier status in II3, as explained earlier in this chapter (p. 123).

Further Reading

Crow, J.F. (2000). The origins, patterns and implications of human spontaneous mutation. *Nature Reviews Genetics*, **1**, 40–47.

Youssoufian, H. and Pyeritz, R.E. (2002). Mechanisms and consequences of somatic mosaicism in humans. *Nature Reviews Genetics*, **3**, 748–758.

Zlotogora, J. (1998). Germline mosaicism. *Human Genetics*, **102**, 381–386.

7

Polygenic and Multifactorial Inheritance

In previous chapters, attention has focused on risk calculation in single-gene disorders. In this chapter, we shall consider how to approach the difficult task of estimating risks for the large number of human characteristics and diseases that clearly have an underlying genetic component but that do not conform to any obvious pattern of straightforward Mendelian inheritance. Many human characteristics are probably determined by the interaction of many genes acting in concert, with each contributing in a small additive way to the overall phenotype. A characteristic determined in this way is said to show *polygenic inheritance.* Similarly, there are many diseases that show familial clustering with incidence figures in close relatives that are considerably less than would be expected if the conditions in question were caused by mutations in single genes. Examples are found in all age groups and include many relatively common congenital malformations, such as spina bifida and cleft lip/palate, plus acquired disorders of later life such as late-onset Alzheimer's disease, insulin-dependent diabetes mellitus, and schizophrenia. These disorders are generally referred to as showing *multifactorial inheritance.*

It should be stated at the outset that these concepts, particularly that of multifactorial inheritance, are not well understood and await clarification at the molecular level. Progress has been achieved for some disorders, most notably Hirschsprung's disease (McCabe, 2002). In this condition there is accumulating evidence that, in at least some families, the proto-oncogene, *RET*, is a major susceptibility locus, with heterozygous mutations identified in around 50% of all familial cases. Mutations in at least nine other genes involved in *RET*-related pathways can also play a role. Consequently, Hirschsprung's disease has been described as showing *oligogenic* inheritance and is often quoted as the model for the study of the so-called common diseases. However, at the time of writing, none of these conditions has been well characterized at the molecular level, and progress in understanding how susceptibility loci interact has been disappointingly slow.

This means that in practice, the geneticist faces a difficult task when counseling an individual or family with a multifactorial disorder. The simplest approach is to use empiric risk data derived locally or in a comparable population. If such data are not available, then calculated risk estimates can be employed, as outlined in the following pages.

7.1 Polygenic Inheritance and the Normal Distribution

Many human characteristics show a continuous distribution, with most individuals having values that fall near the middle of the range. Examples include growth parameters such as height and head circumference, as well as other features such as blood pressure, skin color, and intelligence. The distribution observed for each of these characteristics closely resembles that of a normal (Gaussian) curve. This takes the form of a symmetrical bell-shaped curve distributed evenly about a mean. The spread of the distribution about the mean is determined by the standard deviation.

It is possible to show that a characteristic with a normal distribution in the general population can be generated by polygenic inheritance involving the action of several genes at different loci, each of which makes a small additive contribution to the overall phenotype. As the number of loci increases, the distribution comes to resemble that of a normal curve. Support for the concept that characteristics such as height are determined by the additive effects of many genes at different loci comes from the study of familial correlations. A *correlation* (usually denoted by *r*) is a statistical measure of the degree of association between variable phenomena or, more simply, a measure of the degree of resemblance or relationship between two parameters. As first-degree relatives share on average 50% of their genes, the correlation between first-degree relatives for a polygenic characteristic should be close to 0.5. For characteristics determined exclusively by polygenes (e.g., finger ridge count) this relationship holds true. For other characteristics, such as height, in which environment also plays a role, the correlation between first-degree relatives tends to be somewhat less than 0.5. The proportion of the total phenotypic variance caused by additive genetic variance is called *heritability* and is equal to *r* for identical twins, 2*r* for first-degree relatives, 4*r* for second-degree relatives, and 8*r* for third-degree relatives.

In practice, it is unusual for a genetic counselor to be asked to predict the probable value of a continuous variable characteristic in a future child. In the event that such a request is made, the following approach is suggested. This is illustrated using adult height as an example, this being the human characteristic that has been studied most carefully.

Galton, in his original studies of human variation, showed that the average height of offspring tends to fall slightly closer to the mean population value than to the midparental height. (The midparental height equals the average height of the parents corrected for sex.) This is illustrated diagrammatically in Figure 7.1. If height shows true exclusive polygenic inheritance, then it would be expected that the measurements in offspring would be distributed evenly around the mean of

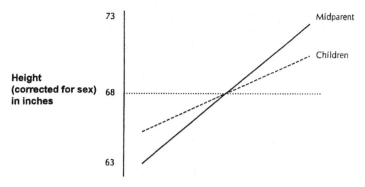

Figure 7.1. The average height of children tends to lie closer to the mean than to the average height of their parents. This example of regression to the mean was first demonstrated by Francis Galton, a cousin of Charles Darwin.

their parents' values. The fact that the average height of offspring tends to revert slightly to the population average (*regression to the mean*) indicates that other factors, such as environment and possibly also dominant genes, play a role. It can be shown (Falconer and Mackay, 1996) that the regression of mean offspring value on the midparent value equals the heritability. Mathematically, this can be depicted as

$$y = \bar{y} + h^2(x - \bar{x})$$

where

y = mean offspring height

x = midparental height

$\bar{y}$ = mean offspring height in population

$\bar{x}$ = mean parental height in population (in practice, $\bar{y} = \bar{x}$)

h^2 = heritability

Therefore, if a value can be obtained for heritability in the relevant population, it is possible to predict the average height of a child born to any couple based on knowledge of their corrected midparental height and the average height of the general population. Stated more simply, the expected height of a child equals the population mean plus the difference between the parents' mean and the population mean multiplied by the heritability.

Example

A healthy couple of above-average height wish to know the probable average height of their future children. The man is 190 cm (75 in.) tall and his partner is 175 cm (69 in.) tall. The female partner's height corrected for sex equals $175 \times 1.08 = 189$ cm. Therefore, the corrected midparental height $= 189.5$ cm. The couple come from a population in which the heritability for height equals approximately 0.8. The average height of the population, corrected for sex, equals 176.5 cm.

The average height of offspring can be calculated from the regression equation

$$y = \bar{y} + h^2(x - \bar{x})$$

where

$$y = \text{mean offspring height}$$
$$\bar{y} = \text{mean height of population} = \bar{x}$$
$$x = \text{midparental height}$$
$$h^2 = \text{heritability} = 0.8$$

Therefore

$$y = 176.5 + 0.8\ (189.5 - 176.5)$$
$$= 186.9 \text{ cm}$$

This value of 186.9 cm (73.6 in.) is the predicted average height for sons. The value for daughters equals $186.9 \div 1.08 = 173$ cm (68.1 in). Note that these are average values. The actual offspring heights will be distributed symmetrically around these average values.

Key Point 1

For a continuous polygenic characteristic, the average value in offspring equals the population mean plus the difference between the parents' mean and the population mean multiplied by the heritability, i.e.,

$$y = \bar{y} + h^2(x - \bar{x})$$

7.2 The Liability/Threshold Model

Traditionally, multifactorial inheritance is believed to involve the interaction of environmental factors with an innate susceptibility determined by the additive effects of many genes. Several ingenious hypotheses and models have been proposed to explain the likely underlying genesis of these disorders. These models have usually been based on the assumption that the disorder represents the "visible" tail end or extreme of an underlying characteristic believed to show a normal distribution curve in the general population. Discontinuity of the phenotype (i.e., affected or unaffected) is explained by superimposition of a threshold beyond which morphogenesis or homeostasis goes awry.

Credit for the *heritability of liability* model is attributed to Falconer (1965), who generously acknowledged that his thoughts owed much to the original studies on pyloric stenosis undertaken by Carter (1961). This model proposes that all of the factors, genetic and environmental, that influence the presence or absence of a multifactorial disease can be considered as a single entity known as *liability*. The liabilities of individuals in a population form a continuous variable. The distinction between affected and unaffected is generated by a threshold at a particular level of liability. If it is assumed that liability in the general population shows a normal distribution, then, although liability of an individual cannot be measured, the mean liability of a group can be determined from the incidence of the disease in that group using statistics of the normal distribution. The units of measurement are therefore standard deviations, and these can be used to estimate the correlation between relatives. This, in turn, enables the genetic (polygenic) contribution to variance of liability (i.e., the heritability) to be determined.

Modifications of this model were proposed by Reich et al. (1972) and by Morton and Maclean (1974). According to Reich et al., there could be different thresholds for different degrees of a disorder or for each sex. Morton and Maclean devised a mixed model to allow for the action of a major gene, a polygenic background, and an environmental component. This was developed by Lalouel et al. (1977) in relation to pyloric stenosis. Finally, mention should be made of the *tetrachorial* model expounded by Edwards (1969) based on the bivariate distribution of the genotypic values between two related individuals.

Each of these models can be developed to derive recurrence risks for family members (Curnow, 1972; Lange et al., 1976). The mathematical principles involved are usually formidable, and in practice it is much easier to resort to empiric data, as already indicated. When empiric data are not available the following guidelines (Section 7.3), together with computer-generated risks (Section 7.4), can be used.

Key Point 2

Falconer's liability/threshold model proposes that a population's genetic and environmental susceptibility, known collectively as *liability*, is normally distributed. An individual is affected if his or her liability lies beyond a threshold superimposed on the liability curve.

7.3 General Principles in Counseling for Multifactorial Disorders

A number of factors can influence the recurrence risk in multifactorial disorders. If possible, these should be considered and, if appropriate, taken into account when counseling. These factors are listed below and illustrated using data obtained in a family study of cleft lip with and without cleft palate undertaken by Carter et al. (1982).

1. *The severity of the disorder.* If the proband is very severely affected, then risks to close relatives are greater than if the proband is only mildly affected. In the cleft lip and palate study, the incidence in siblings was 1.9% if the proband had unilateral cleft lip but rose to 6.6% if the proband had bilateral cleft lip and palate.
2. *The relationship to the proband.* The recurrence risk is greatest among close relatives and decreases rapidly with distance of relationship. The incidence of facial clefting in the offspring and siblings of probands was 3.15% and 2.79%, respectively, compared with much lower values of 0.47% and 0.27% for second- and third-degree relatives.
3. *The number of affected individuals in the family.* If there is more than one affected close relative, then risks for other relatives are increased. For facial clefting, if two siblings are affected, then the risk to a subsequent sibling is approximately 10%. If a parent and a child are affected, then the risk to another child is approximately 14%.
4. *The sex of the proband.* If the disorder in question is more common in one sex, there is a tendency for recurrence risks to be greater for relatives of the less commonly affected sex. In the study of Carter et al. (1982), index patients showed a male:female ratio of approximately 2:1. The recurrence risks for siblings of male and female probands were 2.7% and 3.4%, respectively.
5. *Consanguinity.* It can be shown that with consanguinity, the distribution of liability in the consanguineous population will have a higher variance than in the population in general. In simple terms, this means that the normal curve will be broader and flatter, so that the area falling beyond the threshold becomes greater. Multifactorial disorders therefore show a slightly increased incidence in the offspring of consanguineous matings, although this is not nearly as striking as for autosomal recessive disorders.

In general, the recurrence risk for multifactorial disorders will be slightly greater for consanguineous parents than for those who are unrelated. Bonaiti (1978) produced a graph showing the relative increase in risk of cleft palate for different parental coefficients of inbreeding given different affected relatives. For first cousins (coefficient of relationship $= R = 1/8$) who have had one child with a cleft palate, there is a relative risk of approximately 1.15 for recurrence compared with that of unrelated parents. Therefore, if unrelated parents who have had one child with cleft palate are given a 3% recurrence risk for their next child, then if the parents are first cousins this risk will rise to $3 \times 1.15 = 3.45\%$ If they have had two affected children, the relative risk will be 1.05, i.e., 1.05 times the risk given to unrelated parents.

For second-cousin parents ($R = 1/32$) the relative risk will be less than 1.05 and so effectively can be ignored. If one of the consanguineous parents is affected, then the relative risk rises considerably to approximately 1.25 for first cousins and 1.10 for second cousins. The highest relative risk occurs when a relative on the pathway of relationship is affected. For example, if a paternal grandparent is affected, this will lead to a threefold increase in relative risk for the offspring of first cousins. Note, however, that this will still represent a low risk, as this paternal grandparent will only be a second-degree relative of the person at risk. The values given above are approximate and are appropriate only for cleft palate. Nevertheless, they illustrate the general principles involved and demonstrate that in most instances consanguinity does not make a major difference to recurrence risks for multifactorial disorders.

Key Point 3

Factors that can influence the recurrence risk for multifactorial disorders include the severity of the disorder in the proband, the relationship to the proband, the number of affected persons in the family, the sex of the proband, and parental consanguinity.

7.4 Computer Program for Risk Estimation

Ideally, empiric risks should be used when counseling for multifactorial disorders. Preferably the data should have been collected in a population showing a similar incidence and sharing the same environment as the consultand. This is particularly important for conditions such as neural tube defects, which show strikingly different geographical and ethnic frequencies. Reference should therefore always be made to the standard textbooks on genetic counseling and relevant contemporary literature when presented with a family seeking information about recurrence risks for a multifactorial disorder.

In practice, situations can arise for which no empiric risk information can be obtained. To deal with this eventuality, Charles Smith (1971 and 1972) devised a computer program, RISKMF, with which recurrence risks could be estimated using knowledge of the population incidence and the heritability of the condition. This program can incorporate information on affected and unaffected relatives along with sex or age effects on incidence. For those who are mathematically minded, the method used to estimate recurrence risks depends on "partitioning the genetic distribution of liability into a number of classes, estimating the risk in each class, and numerically integrating over all classes" (Smith, 1971).

Recurrence risks derived using this computer program for various family structures, given different population frequencies and heritability values, are presented in Table 7.1. Risk tables dealing specifically with cleft lip with and without cleft palate, pyloric stenosis, and neural tube defects have been published elsewhere (Bonaiti-Pellié and Smith, 1974). Use of Table 7.1 is relatively straightforward. If, for example, a consultand presents with a history of schizophrenia (population frequency 1%, heritability 80%) in one parent and one sibling, then a risk of 18.7% would be appropriate.

This table is particularly valuable if multiple family members are affected, as empiric risks are not always available for these situations. It is notable that if two parents are affected, risks are much higher than for two affected siblings, since parents are genetically unrelated. For example, the child of two schizophrenic parents has a risk of 40.3%, whereas the brother or sister of two affected siblings with healthy parents runs a risk of only 14.6%.

Table 7.1. Recurrence Risks in Multifactorial Inheritance (%)

Population Frequency (%)	Heritability (%)	Affected Parents								
		0			1			2		
		Affected Siblings								
		0	1	2	0	1	2	0	1	2
	80	0.9	6.7	14.6	8.5	18.7	27.9	40.3	45.9	50.6
1.0	60	1.0	4.9	10.6	5.7	12.3	19.2	21.7	28.3	34.1
	40	1.0	3.3	6.5	3.5	7.0	11.2	9.7	14.1	18.7
	80	0.5	5.1	12.3	6.2	15.5	24.3	37.6	43.2	47.9
0.5	60	0.5	3.4	8.4	3.8	9.5	15.8	18.1	24.4	30.0
	40	0.5	2.1	4.7	2.2	4.9	8.3	7.0	10.8	14.9
	80	0.1	2.6	8.4	2.9	9.8	17.6	30.4	36.7	41.2
0.1	60	0.1	1.5	4.6	1.5	5.0	9.6	11.5	17.1	22.2
	40	0.1	0.7	2.2	0.7	2.2	4.2	3.6	6.0	8.7

Source: Data obtained using the RISKMF computer program (Smith, 1972) reproduced with permission of Dr. Charles Smith and provided by Dr. Susan Holloway.

Unfortunately, Table 7.1 does not permit affected second- or third-degree relatives to be taken into account, although this can be achieved using the RISKMF program. Smith (1971) concluded that "as a rough guide," two affected second-degree relatives or several third-degree relatives will be equivalent to one affected first-degree relative. Degrees of relationship have been considered in Chapter 3 and are summarized in Table 7.2. When undertaking this exercise, remember that the degree of relationship relates to the individual at risk, who will often be an unborn baby. For example, a woman who has had two sisters with spina bifida may wish to know the risk that her baby might be affected. This baby will have two affected second-degree relatives, who, according to Smith, will be roughly equivalent to one affected first-degree relative.

If only a single second- or third-degree relative is affected, the risk contributed by this individual can be estimated using the approach outlined by Edwards (1976).

Table 7.2. Degrees of Relationship

	Proportion of Genes Shared	Relationship
First	$\frac{1}{2}$	Parents, children, siblings
Second	$\frac{1}{4}$	Uncles/aunts, nephews/nieces, grand-parents, grandchildren, half-siblings
Third	$\frac{1}{8}$	First cousins, great-grandparents, great-grandchildren, half-uncles/aunts, half-nephews/nieces

This is based on the assumption that the correlation between relatives is halved for each degree of relationship. The incidence in first- (I_1), second- (I_2), and third- (I_3) degree relatives, given a population incidence of P, has been shown by Edwards to be

$$I_1 = \sqrt{P} = P^{1/2}$$
$$I_2 = \sqrt{I_1 \times P} = (I_1 \times P)^{1/2} = P^{3/4}$$
$$I_3 = \sqrt{\sqrt{I_1 \times P^3}} = \sqrt{\sqrt{P^{3.5}}} = P^{7/8}$$

Therefore, for cleft lip with or without cleft palate with a population frequency of 1 in 1000, the incidence in first-, second-, and third-degree relatives will be 0.03 (1 in 30), 0.005 (1 in 200), and 0.002 (1 in 500), respectively. These figures can be used as rough estimates of maximum risk if only one member of a family is affected. If more than one member of a family is affected, with, for example, one affected first-degree relative plus one affected second-degree relative, then it is very difficult to derive recurrence risks without access to carefully collected empiric data or the RISKMF program. It should be noted that the sum of the risks contributed by each affected relative will generally underestimate the true risk, particularly if the affected individuals are themselves not related by blood.

Key Point 4

If suitable empiric data are not available, recurrence risks can be obtained using the RISKMF computer program; for example, see Table 7.1. Alternatively, risks can be estimated using the formulae $I_1 = P^{1/2}$, $I_2 = P^{3/4}$, and $I_3 = P^{7/8}$.

7.5 The Use of Susceptibility Loci

Most of the single-gene disorders encountered at a genetics clinic have now been characterized at the molecular level. Consequently, the focus of research in molecular genetics has started to switch to polygenic/multifactorial disease, with the short-term goal of identifying loci that convey susceptibility to the more common acquired disorders of adult life. The identification of a polymorphic marker or locus showing a strong association with a particular disease raises the possibility that this can be used for predictive purposes, both in affected families and in the general population. To date the practical applications of this approach have been very limited, but this situation is starting to change as more powerful methods of detecting linkage and association are developed in parallel with the information gained from the Human Genome Project. Several commercial companies now offer "predictive genomic profiling" for common conditions such as Alzheimer's disease, coronary artery disease, and osteoporosis based on recent reports of alleged disease associations, some of which have proved to be more robust than others. In contrast, most professional bodies representing human and medical geneticists have expressed unease that these new discoveries are being exploited for commercial purposes before their validity and clinical role have been established. The controversy surrounding the use of susceptibility loci in a clinical setting will be illustrated using ankylosing spondylitis and Alzheimer's disease, these being examples of multifactorial disorders for which strong associations have been established.

Ankylosing Spondylitis

Ankylosing spondylitis (AS) shows a very strong association with the HLA-B27 allele. Approximately 95% of all white patients with AS are B27-positive, in contrast to the general population frequency of B27 of roughly 10%. The general population incidence of clinical symptomatic AS is approximately 0.1%.

Predictive Testing in the General Population

The precise probability that any B27-positive member of the general population will develop AS can be determined by carrying out a simple Bayesian calculation (Table 7.3), which yields a risk of 0.94%. Conversely, 99.06% of B27-positive individuals will not develop AS. Using a similar calculation, it can be shown that the probability that a B27-negative individual will develop AS equals 0.0000556 or 1 in 17,883 (Table 7.4). Approximate values for these probabilities can be calculated more easily by considering a population of 100,000, in which 10,000 will be B27-positive. This population will contain 100 people with AS, 95 of whom will be B27-positive. Therefore, the probability that a B27-positive member of the population will have AS equals approximately 95/10,000 or 0.95%. (Note that these two methods give slightly different answers, depending on whether the B27 frequency of 10% applies to only the unaffected population, as in the Bayesian method, or to the total population, as in the quicker method.)

It is worth noting that if the disease in question has a much higher incidence, then the disease association will have a much greater predictive value. For example,

Table 7.3.

Probability	Affected with AS	Not Affected with AS
Prior	0.001	0.999
Conditional		
B27-positive	0.95	0.1
Joint	0.00095	0.0999
Posterior probability		

$$\text{Affected} = \frac{0.00095}{0.00095 + 0.0999} = 0.0094$$

$$\text{Not affected} = \frac{0.0999}{0.00095 + 0.0999} = 0.9906$$

AS, ankylosing spondylitis.

Table 7.4.

Probability	Affected with AS	Not Affected with AS
Prior	0.001	0.999
Conditional		
B27 negative	0.05	0.9
Joint	0.00005	0.8991
Posterior probability		

$$\text{Affected} = \frac{0.00005}{0.00005 + 0.8991} = 0.0000556$$

$$\text{Not affected} = \frac{0.8991}{0.00005 + 0.8991} = 0.9999444$$

AS, ankylosing spondylitis.

for a disease with an incidence of 1%, such as schizophrenia, a marker present in 95% of patients but only 10% of the population will convey a risk of approximately 9% for developing the disease.

Modifying Risks in Families

In general, AS is believed to be a multifactorial disorder with an empiric risk of around 5% that the offspring of an affected parent will develop clinical disease (Emery and Lawrence, 1967). The actual risks differ, depending on the sex of the proband and offspring, but for the purposes of this discussion, these differences will be ignored. Following the discovery of the strong B27 association, it was suggested that B27 testing could be used to modify this prior risk for offspring of 1 in 20 (Falace et al., 1978). This suggestion was opposed on the grounds that testing of offspring could introduce a risk of "iatrogenic HLA-B27-itis," and because of this possibility, it has been proposed that the problems are such that B27 typing "is not justified" (Gran and Husby, 1995).

To this ethical concern can be added the practical difficulty of knowing how best to modify the offspring risk mathematically, which in turn relates directly to the prevailing limited understanding of the genetic and physiological relationship between AS and the B27 allele. While it is true that this is one of the strongest known disease associations, it is important to remember that only 1% of B27-positive individuals develop AS and 5% of affected individuals are B27-negative. This limited understanding is further illustrated by the observation that homozygosity for B27 does not confer increased susceptibility. Furthermore, the MZ:DZ twin concordance rates of 60%:12% emphasize the important role played by other unknown genetic and environmental factors (Wordsworth and Brown, 1997).

A practical compromise often adopted is to double the empiric risk of 5% to 10% if a child inherits the high-risk B27 allele. A B27-positive adult with AS will transmit the B27 allele to on average 50% of his children. Thus, if he has 100 children, 50 will be B27-positive and 5 of these will develop AS, assuming, as is likely, that all of the children who develop clinical disease will be B27-positive—hence the 10% risk. The likelihood that a B27-negative offspring will be affected is very low and almost certainly less than 1%.

Late-Onset Alzheimer's Disease

In contrast to early "presenile" Alzheimer's disease, the common late-onset form, which shows an exponential rise in incidence after the age of 65 years, is believed to show multifactorial inheritance. Linkage and association studies indicate that at least five loci are involved, with the apolipoprotein E (APOE) locus making a major contribution. The frequency of the APOE ε4 allele is significantly increased in affected patients (56%) in comparison with controls (24%). This observation has led to the offer of APOE ε4 testing for members of the general population who are understandably concerned that the onset of Alzheimer's disease will shorten their lives and blight their retirement.

By applying the same type of Bayesian calculation used for AS (Tables 7.3 and 7.4), lifetime risks for developing Alzheimer's disease have been developed based on the presence of zero, one, or two APOE ε4 alleles (Liddell et al., 2001; Seshadri et al., 1995). Table 7.5 illustrates the basic principle. At age 65 years, the lifetime risk of developing Alzheimer's disease has been shown in epidemiological studies to be approximately 15% (0.15). Using this as the prior risk and the aforementioned values of 56% and 24% for the frequencies of APOE ε4 in Alzheimer patients and controls as conditional probabilities, it can be shown that at age 65 years, the lifetime risk of developing the disease increases to 29% for those with an APOE ε4 allele and falls to 9% for those without this allele (Table 7.5). More detailed risks derived using this approach are given in Table 7.6.

Proponents of population susceptibility testing argue that knowledge of these risks allows individuals to plan their lives accordingly. Critics make the reasonable point that it is not possible to predict the age of onset and that even those deemed to be at highest risk (i.e., APOE ε4 female homozygotes) have a close to 50% chance

Table 7.5.

Probability	Lifetime Risk of Developing AD	Lifetime Risk of Not Developing AD
Prior	0.15	0.85
Conditional		
APOE ε4-positive	0.56	0.24
Joint	0.084	0.204

Posterior probability of developing AD for a 65-year-old who is APOE ε4-positive $= 0.084/(0.084 + 0.204) = 0.29$

Posterior probability of not developing AD for a 65-year-old who is APOE ε4-positive $= 0.204/(0.084 + 0.204) = 0.71$

AD, late-onset Alzheimer's disease.

Table 7.6. Lifetime Risk of Developing Late-Onset
Alzheimer's Disease for a 65-Year-Old According to
Gender and APOE ε4 Status

APOE ε4 Status	Male (%)	Female (%)
Unknown	6.3	12
Negative	4.6	9.3
Heterozygote	12	23
Homozygote	35	53

Source: Reproduced with permission from Liddell et al. (2001).

of not developing the disease. These concerns have prompted several influential bodies, including Alzheimer's Disease International, the American College of Medical Genetics and Society of Human Genetics, and the Alzheimer's Association to conclude that APOE genotyping has no role in prediction or risk assessment.

The extent to which risks conveyed by a family history of Alzheimer's disease are influenced by APOE testing is not clear, with various studies giving conflicting results (Huang et al., 2004). Some studies have indicated that the APOE ε4 allele does contribute to familial risks, possibly by influencing age of onset, but at present the evidence is not sufficiently robust to allow familial risks to be modified.

Key Point 5

At present, the use of susceptibility loci and disease associations in multifactorial disease is extremely limited, partly because of widespread ethical concern about causing undue anxiety and partly because of the lack of understanding of the mechanisms involved.

Further Reading

Falconer, D.S. and Mackay, T.F.C. (1996). *Introduction to quantitative genetics.* Longman, Harlow.

King, R.A., Rotter, J.I., and Motulsky, A.G. (eds.). (2002). *The genetic basis of common diseases*, 2nd ed. Oxford University Press, Oxford.

McGuffin, P., Owen, M.J., and Gottesman, I.I. (eds.). (2002). *Psychiatric genetics and genomics.* Oxford University Press, Oxford.

8

Cancer Genetics

It is now well established that genetic factors play an important role in causing cancer. In most cases, the causal mutations are not inherited but are acquired somatically, possibly as part of the normal aging process or as a result of prolonged exposure to particular carcinogens. In these situations, any observed small increase in risk to close family relatives is just as likely to be due to shared environmental exposure as to an inherited germline susceptibility. However, in up to 5% of cases of the common cancers, notably breast and colorectal cancers, there is evidence for a strong inherited susceptibility. This is generally attributed to single-gene inheritance, possibly influenced by other modifying genes and low-penetrance alleles. Multifactorial inheritance, implying the interaction of additive *polygenes* with the environment, probably plays a role in a further 10%–20% of cases. In addition, several single-gene disorders have been identified in which particular cancers show a high incidence. Recognition of these high-risk cancer families and familial cancer syndromes is important because of the potential for early detection and treatment through appropriate screening.

Increasing awareness of familial susceptibility to common cancers and the existence of high-risk familial cancer-predisposing syndromes has led to the widespread introduction of cancer genetics clinics at which the assessment of an individual's risk for developing a particular cancer is an integral component. To some extent, risk assessment in cancer genetics can be viewed as more of an art than a science, as limited understanding of the basic mechanisms involved often precludes precise risk determination. Thus, the priority in most situations is to undertake risk assessment or estimation, rather than a precise risk calculation, with a view to categorizing an individual's risk as high, moderate, or low. This, in turn, leads to an offer of appropriate screening and intervention. In this chapter, the basic principles involved will be illustrated using breast and colorectal cancer as examples, as these are the two most common forms of cancer that prompt referral to cancer genetics clinics.

8.1 Breast Cancer

Breast cancer is the most common form of cancer in women, with a lifetime incidence in the Western world of approximately 10%. Factors believed to be associated with an increased risk include nulliparity, absence of breast-feeding, early menarche, obesity, alcohol ingestion, and the use of hormone replacement therapy. In addition, a positive family history is of major importance, an observation that has prompted the development of several models for risk prediction based exclusively on this parameter.

Models for Predicting Breast Cancer Risk

The Claus Model

The first and still most widely applied method for estimating breast cancer risk is based on a large epidemiological survey known as the Cancer and Steroid Hormone (CASH) study. This involved analysis of 4730 confirmed breast cancer cases matched with 4688 controls (Claus et al., 1990). These women were not selected because of a known positive family history. The incidence of breast cancer in the first-degree relatives of the probands was found to be double that in the first-degree relatives of the controls. Based on detailed analysis of the family histories of the index cases and controls, and assuming an autosomal dominant gene model with reduced penetrance, tables were drawn up giving age-specific risks for a woman with one or two close relatives affected with breast cancer at various ages of onset (Claus et al., 1994). Two examples are shown in Tables 8.1 and 8.2, which indicate the cumulative probability of breast cancer for a woman who has one or two affected first-degree relatives. In these tables, it can be seen that the probability that a woman will develop breast cancer by age 79 years is 0.21 if she has one first-degree relative who was affected between the ages of 20 and 29 years, and 0.46 if she has another first-degree relative affected between the ages of 30 and 39 years. These CASH or Claus data sets are now used extensively when estimating risks for developing breast

Table 8.1. Predicted Cumulative Probability of Breast Cancer for a Woman Who Has One First-Degree Relative Affected with Breast Cancer

Age of Woman (yrs)	First-Degree Relative with Age of Onset (yrs)					
	20–29	30–39	40–49	50–59	60–69	70–79
29	.007	.005	.003	.002	.002	.001
39	.025	.017	.012	.008	.006	.005
49	.062	.044	.032	.023	.018	.015
59	.116	.086	.064	.049	.040	.035
69	.171	.130	.101	.082	.070	.062
79	.211	.165	.132	.110	.096	.088

Table 8.2. Predicted Cumulative Probability of Breast Cancer for a Women Who has Two First-Degree Relatives Affected With Breast Cancer, By Age of Onset of the Affected Relatives

Age of Onset of First Relative (yr)										
	20–29						30–39			
Age of Onset of Second Relative (yr)										
Age (yr)	20–29	30–39	40–49	50–59	60–69	70–79	30–39	40–49	50–59	60–69	70–79
29	.021	.020	.018	.016	.014	.012	.018	.016	.014	.012	.009
39	.069	.066	.061	.055	.048	.041	.062	.056	.048	.040	.032
49	.166	.157	.146	.133	.117	.099	.148	.134	.116	.096	.077
59	.295	.279	.261	.238	.210	.179	.265	.239	.209	.175	.143
69	.412	.391	.366	.335	.297	.256	.371	.337	.296	.251	.207
79	.484	.460	.434	.397	.354	.308	.437	.399	.353	.302	.252

Age of Onset of First Relative (yr)									
	40–49				50–59			60–69		70–79
Age of Onset of Second Relative (yr)									
Age (yr)	40–49	50–59	60–69	70–79	50–59	60–69	70–79	60–69	70–79	70–79
29	.014	.012	.009	.007	.009	.006	.005	.004	.003	.002
39	.048	.039	.030	.023	.030	.022	.016	.016	.012	.008
49	.117	.096	.075	.058	.075	.056	.042	.041	.030	.023
59	.210	.174	.139	.108	.138	.105	.081	.080	.061	.049
69	.298	.249	.202	.161	.200	.157	.124	.122	.098	.081
79	.354	.300	.246	.200	.245	.195	.158	.156	.128	.109

Source: From *Cancer*, vol. 73, p. 646. Copyright © 1994 American Cancer Society. Reprinted with permission of John Wiley & Sons, Inc.

cancer and can also be used to incorporate a family history of ovarian cancer (Claus et al., 1993).

The Claus data have the virtues of simplicity and widespread availability. However, they do not take into account more than two affected close relatives or information provided by unaffected relatives. Intuitively, it is apparent that a woman whose mother and only sister have breast cancer almost certainly faces a much greater risk than a woman in the same situation who also has a large number of unaffected aunts and sisters. This intuition has been quantified by Schmidt et al. (1998). For a woman with two first-degree relatives who both developed breast cancer at age 45 years, the Claus model predicts a lifetime risk for developing breast cancer of 35%. However, if this woman also has four unaffected maternal aunts and seven unaffected sisters, then her risk of developing breast cancer falls to 8.6%, i.e., less than the general population risk. The Claus data also have the disadvantage that the results of mutation testing cannot be taken into account. This can yield risks as high as 80% (see below). Thus, the Claus model is extremely useful for providing a quick risk assessment for a woman with a very simple family history, which conveys a low prior probability but is of limited value in more complex or higher-risk situations.

Models for Predicting the Likelihood
of a Mutation in *BRCA1/2*

The discovery of two high-penetrance breast and ovarian susceptibility genes (*BRCA1/2*) has prompted the development of several models for estimating the probability that a mutation will be identified in an affected individual. Based on the analysis of families with at least four cases of breast cancer diagnosed below 60 years of age, it has been estimated that approximately 80% of hereditary breast/ovarian cancer families can be attributed to mutations in *BRCA1* and 15% to mutations in *BRCA2*. For breast cancer-only families, the proportions are lower (28% for *BRCA1* and 37% for *BRCA2*) (Ford et al., 1998). The detection rate for mutations in families with fewer affected members is much poorer. Mutations in *BRCA1* are also known to convey significant risks for ovarian cancer, whereas mutations in *BRCA2* show a positive association with breast cancer in males. These observations have been incorporated in the various models to derive prior probabilities that a particular family will harbor a mutation.

The Couch Model

This model was based originally on *BRCA1* testing in 169 women with breast cancer who had a positive family history (Couch et al., 1997) and was subsequently updated to include both *BRCA1* and *BRCA2* analysis in a much larger sample (Blackwood et al., 2001). A mutation in *BRCA1* was identified in 16% of the women. Logistic regression analysis was applied to identify associations between family patterns and the presence or absence of a mutation. Positive predictive factors included early age of onset, multiple primary tumors, ovarian cancer, and Ashkenazi Jewish ancestry. (It is now known that three relatively common founder mutations, two in *BRCA1* and one in *BRCA2*, contribute close to 60% of high-risk Ashkenazi Jewish families.) Disadvantages of the Couch model are that the estimates are based on relatively small numbers and have to be extrapolated for unaffected family members.

The Frank Models

These models are based on the results of mutation analysis undertaken by Myriad Genetics, which holds the patents for *BRCA1/2* gene testing. The first Frank model was developed based on the results of mutation testing in 238 women with breast cancer diagnosed before the age of 50 years, or ovarian cancer at any age, who also had at least one first- or second-degree affected relative (Frank et al., 1998). As with the Couch model, logistic regression analysis was used to identify predictive factors, which included early age of onset, ovarian cancer, and bilateral tumors. Disadvantages of this model are that it cannot be used for women with disease onset after the age of 50 years and that it tends to yield relatively high risks because it was based on known high-risk affected families. An updated version of the Myriad Genetics data (Frank et al., 2002) used a much larger sample size, but with less clear criteria for testing. In addition, as with the first Frank model, data are not provided for women over 50 years of age.

The BRCAPRO Model

This rather complex computer-based model takes into account a woman's affected first- and second-degree relatives, as well as unaffected relatives, to determine the probability that she is a carrier of a *BRCA1/2* mutation (Parmigiani et al., 1998). The analysis is based on large high-risk families and therefore tends to yield relatively high individual risk estimates. This model has been validated (Berry et al., 2002), but its application requires access to the computer program and is therefore time-consuming and impractical in a clinic setting.

The Manchester Model

A relatively simple empiric scoring system for the prediction of pathogenic *BRCA1/2* mutations has been developed based on analysis of families attending cancer genetics clinics in Manchester and Southampton (Evans et al., 2004). Each family contained at least two close relatives who had developed breast cancer before the age of 50 years. The families were analyzed separately as three subsets for the purpose of validation. The scoring system is summarized in Table 8.3. Scores are assigned depending upon the type of cancer and age of onset. A score of 10 is equivalent to a 10% chance of identifying a mutation in *BRCA1* or *BRCA2*, this

Table 8.3. Scoring System for the Likelihood of Identifying a *BRCA1* or *BRCA2* Mutation Based on Evaluation of Family History*

Type of Cancer	Age at Diagnosis (years)	Score BRCA1	BRCA2
Female breast cancer	< 30	6	5
Female breast cancer	30–39	4	4
Female breast cancer	40–49	3	3
Female breast cancer	50–59	2	2
Female breast cancer	> 59	1	1
Male breast cancer	< 60	5[†]	8
Male breast cancer	> 59	5[†]	5
Ovarian cancer	< 60	8	5[‡]
Ovarian cancer	> 59	5	5[‡]
Pancreatic cancer	Any	0	1
Prostate cancer	< 60	0	2
Prostate cancer	> 59	0	1

*In bilateral disease, each breast cancer is counted separately. Ductal carcinoma in situ (DCIS) is included. Scores should be summed counting each cancer in a direct lineage (i.e. on the same side of the family). The scoring system includes a cutoff at 10 points for each gene. This equates to >10% probability of a pathogenic mutation in *BRCA1* and *BRCA2* individually.
[†]If *BRCA2* already tested.
[‡]If *BRCA1* already tested.

Source: Reproduced from Firth and Hurst (2005) and adapted from Evans (2004).

being deemed to be a realistic threshold for testing, given the expense involved. The authors propose a screening strategy consisting of testing for *BRCA2* first if there is an affected male and for *BRCA1* first if there is a woman with ovarian cancer.

A Practical Approach

Given that there is no precise mathematical model for determining breast cancer risks in most situations, the basic approach usually involves a detailed clinical assessment based initially on analysis of all reported cases of cancer in a three-generation family tree. Information is sought about the type of cancer, age of onset, and possible multiple tumor involvement. Specific points that would point to an inherited form of breast cancer susceptibility are summarized in Table 8.4. Note that these include ethnicity, as certain populations, notably Ashkenazi Jews and those with an Icelandic ancestry, have an increased risk because of founder mutations in *BRCA1/2*. It is recommended practice that all alleged cancer diagnoses should be confirmed through review of hospital records or reference to national cancer registries.

When full family details have been obtained, the family is then triaged by reference to referral guidelines and pathways such as those drawn up by the UK Cancer Family Study Group (Eccles et al., 2000—Table 8.5) or the NHS Institute for Clinical Excellence (NICE at www.nice.org.uk/CG014NICEguideline). Women at only slightly increased risk (<1 in 6 to 1 in 8) are managed in primary care settings with reassurance and guidance on breast awareness and lifestyle. Women at moderately increased risk (approximately 1 in 6 to 1 in 3) are managed in secondary care settings with an offer of annual mammography from age 40 years on. Women deemed to be at high risk (>1 in 3) are referred to specialist cancer genetic clinics (tertiary care) for more detailed risk assessment, annual mammography from age 35 to 40 years on, annual transvaginal ultrasound to detect ovarian cancer if appropriate, and discussion of prophylaxis including possible bilateral mastectomy. *BRCA1/2* testing can be initiated if criteria are met (Table 8.3) as long as DNA can be obtained from an affected family member.

Table 8.4. Features Suggestive of an Inherited Susceptibility to Breast Cancer

Early age of onset in affected relatives

Multiple primary tumors in one individual, e.g., bilateral tumors in paired organs or breast *and* ovarian cancers

Two or more first- or second-degree relatives with breast, ovarian, or prostate cancer on one side of the family

One or more males with breast cancer

Two or more relatives with the same rare cancer, such as sarcoma, consistent with a familial cancer syndrome, e.g., Cowden or Li-Fraumeni syndrome

Ethnicity: Ashkenazi Jewish origin—2.3% have one of three common (*BRCA1/2*) founder mutations
Icelandic origin—1 in 200 carry a specific *BRCA2* mutation

Table 8.5. Criteria for Evaluating a Family History of Breast Cancer

Important Guidance for Using the Table

• Work from the *top of the table down* in assessing risk (risk assigned is then the highest level of risk consistent with the family history)
• **Average age** is a simple arithmetic mean, i.e., a woman with relatives affected at 48 years and 39 years (mean $87/2 = 43.5$ year) falls in the bracket 2 relatives diagnosed at 40–49 years
• **Relative** includes first-degree relative (mother, father, brother, sister, child) and their first-degree relatives. For the purposes of this analysis, female relatives linked through a male are included because the penetrance of breast cancer genes is so much lower in males than in females. A history of breast cancer in a paternal aunt age 39 years and paternal grandmother age 47 years would be equivalent to half the risk of a woman with a mother and maternal aunt or grandmother at an average age of 44 years, assuming that a dominant gene is the underlying cause of the paternal family history
• Affected relatives should be on the same side of the family. If there are relevant cancers on both maternal and paternal sides of the family, evaluate both sides separately. The estimate will then depend on whether either side looks like it might be due to a dominant gene or whether both sides look like isolated cases. Non-genetic approaches to risk estimation (such as the Gail method) may then be more helpful
• A relative with clearly bilateral *breast cancer* (i.e., two primaries) should be viewed as two relatives for simplicity
• A male breast cancer can be counted as a young female (<30 years)
• Figures in square brackets [] refer to the cumulative risk of developing breast cancer over the decade between age 40 and 50 years where early mammography may be appropriate
• Early-onset prostate cancer (and other BRCA1/2 associated cancers) in a male relative may be significant
• Family size is important in assessment of risk, e.g. in very large sibships the significance of 2 affected relatives diagnosed at a 50–60 years is lessened; the maximum risks in the table assume no modifying unaffected relatives

High Risk (>1 in 3 Lifetime Risk) Criteria

• Clearly dominant pattern of early onset breast and/or ovarian cancer with an affected first-degree relative
• First-degree relatives where the pattern is consistent with a diagnosis of Li-Fraumeni syndrome

High/Moderate Risk (>1 in 4 Lifetime Risk) Criteria

• Clearly dominant pattern of breast and/or ovarian cancer with affected 2nd-degree relatives on the paternal side of the family
• First-degree relative with breast and ovarian cancer with age at diagnosis of first cancer <50 years
• 3 relatives diagnosed with breast cancer and/or ovarian cancer, with the breast cancer at average age of 50–60 years (1 in 4 risk) [6–7%]
• 2 relatives (one first-degree) with breast cancer diagnosed <40 years

Moderate Risk (>1 in 6 Lifetime Risk) Criteria

• 2 relatives diagnosed with breast cancer at any age (1 in 4–1 in 6 risk) [4%]
• 1 first-degree relative diagnosed with breast cancer <40 years (maximum 1 in 6 risk) [4%]
• 1 male relative diagnosed with breast cancer at any age (maximum 1 in 6 risk) [3–4%]
• 1 relative with both breast and ovarian cancer (diagnosed at any age)

Slightly Increased Risk (<1 in 6 Lifetime Risk) Criteria

• 1 first-degree or a few distant relatives with no clearly dominant pattern of inheritance and age at onset >50 years
• 1 first-degree relative diagnosed >40 years (assuming negative family history) (1 in 6–1 in 12) [2–3%]

Population Risk (1 in 11 Lifetime Risk) Criterion

• No family history of breast or ovarian cancer and an average environmental risk profile [1%]

Source: Reproduced from Firth and Hurst (2005) and adapted from Eccles et al. (2000).

Risks Based on BRCA1/2 Mutation Analysis

Mutations in *BRCA1/2* show age-related penetrance. Estimated breast and ovarian cancer risks are generally higher in studies based on multiple-case families than in those based on cases that were not selected because of a strong positive family history. This is probably because studies using multiple-case families have been enriched for more pathogenic mutations or because other familial and/or environmental factors are present in these families. Cumulative risks for breast and ovarian cancer to age 70 years for *BRCA1* mutation carriers average around 70%–85% and 45%–60%, respectively, for multiple-case families, whereas average risks of 65% and 40% have been obtained for unselected cases (Antoniou et al., 2003). Comparable risks for *BRCA2* carriers are 60%–85% (breast) and 27%–31% (ovarian) for multiple-case families and 45% (breast) and 11% (ovarian) for unselected cases. Since most women with a *BRCA1/2* mutation who are being counseled will have been ascertained because of a strong positive family history, the higher risk figures are usually more appropriate. Table 8.6 shows average age-dependent cumulative risks, which can be used when the precise mode of ascertainment is uncertain.

Example 1

A 25-year-old woman is referred for *BRCA1* testing following receipt of a letter from her sister, who has undergone *BRCA1* gene testing and been informed that she carries a pathogenic mutation. Details of the family history are unclear. The woman agrees to mutation analysis and is found to be a carrier of the same mutation. She wishes to know the probability that she will develop breast or ovarian cancer at some point in her life. These risks can be read off from Table 8.6 as 74% and 48%, respectively.

Table 8.6. Risk of Cancer by Age in *BRCA1/2* Carriers

Age (years)	Risk (%) in *BRCA1* Carrier of		Risk (%) in *BRCA2* Carrier of	
	Breast Cancer	Ovarian Cancer	Breast Cancer	Ovarian Cancer
25	0	0	0	0
30	2	1	1	0
35	7	2	4	0
40	16	4	7	0
45	30	8	14	0
50	41	15	20	1
55	50	20	26	3
60	55	27	31	5
65	59	33	36	7
70	64	38	49	9
75	69	43	60	11
80	74	48	69	12

Source: Reproduced from Firth and Hurst (2005).

Example 2

A 50-year-old woman with a similar family history is found to carry the *BRCA1* mutation, which has been identified in her sister. She wishes to know the probability that she will develop breast cancer and/or ovarian cancer by age 80 years. Reference to Table 8.6 indicates that by age 50 years, 41% of heterozygotes will have developed breast cancer, leaving 59% unaffected. An additional 33% are affected by age 80 years. Thus, the probability that the 50-year-old woman will develop breast cancer in the next 30 years equals 33/59, which equals 0.56 or 56%. Note that it would be incorrect to quote the cumulative risk of 0.74 or 74% directly from Table 8.6. The probability that this 50-year-old woman will develop ovarian cancer by age 80 years equals 33/85, which equals 0.39 or 39%.

This example illustrates a useful general principle, which can be applied when an unaffected individual who has reached a certain age wishes to know the probability of becoming affected by a specific age in the future. If the cumulative probability of developing disease at the present age (P) equals x and at the future age (F) equals y, then the risk of developing disease between the ages of P and F equals

$$\frac{y - x}{1 - x}$$

Example 3

A 40-year-old woman who is a known *BRCA2* mutation carrier and who has already undergone mastectomy because of a confirmed cancer wishes to know the probability that she will develop another tumor in her remaining breast. Table 8.7 indicates the age-related cumulative probability for developing a second tumor in the contralateral breast for *BRCA1/2* carriers. Using the simple formula $(y - x)/(1 - x)$ derived in the previous example, the probability that this woman will develop a second tumor equals $(0.57 - 0.18)/(1 - 0.18)$, which equals 0.48 or 48%.

Table 8.7. Risk of Developing a Second Contralateral Breast Cancer in a *BRCA1/2* Carrier

Age (years)	Risk (%)	
	BRCA1 Carrier	*BRCA2* Carrier
40	33	18
50	50	37
60	60	48
70	65	52
80	70	57

Source: Reproduced from Firth and Hurst (2005).

Does a Negative *BRCA1/2* Mutation Screen Reduce the Risk of Cancer in a Woman from a High-Risk Family?

If a woman tests negative for a mutation that is present in other family members, then it is almost certainly reasonable to counsel her on the basis that her risk for developing cancer is no greater than that of the general population, with the possible caveat that some high-incidence families may also harbor high-risk modifier genes or other shared adverse environmental factors that could convey a modest increase in risk.

How should an unaffected woman be counseled if her affected relatives have tested negative on *BRCA1/2* screening? It could be argued that if a woman is in a high-risk category and her affected relatives test negative on *BRCA1/2* mutation analysis, then her lifetime risk for developing breast/ovarian cancer is reduced, as the normal *BRCA1/2* mutation screen in her affected relatives has reduced the probability that the family harbors a high-penetrance susceptibility gene. This would be valid if it could be established that all or a large proportion of high-risk category families have a detectable *BRCA1/2* mutation. At present this does not apply, particularly to families with only breast cancer, firstly, because not all mutations can be identified by the mutation scanning techniques presently in use and, secondly, because it is strongly suspected that other breast cancer susceptibility genes are involved in many of these families. The failure to identify a mutation in *BRCA1/2* in an affected individual from a high-risk category family could reflect a chance association of random cases, but it is also possible that the family harbors a high-penetrance allele in another as yet unidentified susceptibility gene. Thus, until the underlying genetic contribution to breast and ovarian cancers is fully elucidated, it is probably wise to resist the temptation to reduce a high risk on the basis of a normal *BRCA1/2* gene test in a close affected relative.

Key Point 1

Risk assessment for women with a family history of breast cancer with or without ovarian cancer generally involves an estimate of risk based on review of the family history, with categorization into high (1 in 3), moderate (1 in 6 to 1 in 3), or low (<1 in 6) risk, depending upon the number of affected relatives and other factors including age of onset, bilateral tumors, combined breast and ovarian cancers, and breast cancer in a male. When the family history fulfills the criteria for genetic testing, *BRCA1/2* mutation analysis should be undertaken. Risks for subsequent development of a tumor or development of a second tumor can be calculated using cumulative risk penetrance figures.

8.2 Colorectal Cancer

Colorectal cancer is one of the most common forms of cancer found in Western communities, with a lifetime incidence of 1 in 18 in males and 1 in 20 in females in the United Kingdom. The nature of the genetic contribution to colorectal cancer is similar to that in breast cancer in that single-gene disorders, such as familial adenomatous polyposis (FAP) and hereditary nonpolyposis colon cancer (HNPCC) together account for approximately 2%–3% of all cases. Genetic susceptibility, probably involving as yet unidentified low-penetrance alleles, plays a role in around 10%–20% of cases. Risk assessment in colorectal cancer is primarily concerned with identifying those families in which there is likely to be a high risk attributable to single-gene inheritance and distinguishing these from the remaining large number of families in which risks can be categorized as moderate or low. Thus, as with breast cancer, the role of the geneticist is to provide an estimate of risk so that appropriate screening and lifestyle advice can be implemented.

Identifying Families at High Risk

Consideration should always be given to the possibility of one of the small number of single-gene disorders that predispose to colorectal cancer. These are FAP, HNPCC, juvenile polyposis, Peutz-Jeghers syndrome, and the recently described autosomal recessive form of polyposis caused by mutations in *MUTYH* (*MYH*). With the exception of HNPCC, these conditions have characteristic phenotypic findings that point to the diagnosis. Because of the lack of distinguishing features in HNPCC, diagnostic criteria have been drawn up based on the family history and the pattern of tumor involvement (Table 8.8).

Once an accurate diagnosis has been established, precise risk estimation can be based on the results of mutation analysis. Occasionally in FAP, no mutation can be identified in an affected relative. In these situations, linkage analysis can be used, as outlined in Chapter 5. If no affected relative is available, risks can be modified based on age-related penetrance (Table 8.9).

Example 4

A 20-year-old man with a strong family history of histologically confirmed FAP wishes to know the probability that he has inherited the condition from his affected father. None of his affected relatives is alive. The man is found to be free of polyps on sigmoidoscopy. From Table 8.9 it can be seen that 80% of individuals with FAP

Table 8.8. Diagnostic Criteria for Hereditary Nonpolyposis Colorectal Cancer (Amsterdam Criteria 2)

There should be at least three relatives on the same side of the family with an
　　HNPCC-associated cancer, i.e., colorectal, endometrial, small bowel, gastric, ovarian,
　　ureter/renal pelvis, hepatobiliary, or skin cancer.
One relative should be a first-degree relative of the other two.
At least two successive generations should be affected.
At least one cancer should be diagnosed before age 50 years.
Familial adenomatous polyposis has been excluded.
Tumors should be verified histologically.

Table 8.9. Probability That Colorectal Polyps
Will Be Identified on Sigmoidoscopy in FAP

Age (years)	Probability (%)
14	40
16	65
18	75
20	80
22	85
24	90
26	91
28	93
30	94
32	95
34	96
36	97
38	98
40	99

FAP, familial adenomatous polyposis.

Source: Data adapted from Burn et al. (1991) and Petersen et al. (1991).

have polyps identifiable on sigmoidoscopy by the age of 20 years. This information can be incorporated in a simple Bayesian calculation, which indicates that the posterior probability that this man has inherited FAP equals 1 in 6 (Table 8.10).

Empiric Risks and Risk Categorisation

Table 8.11 shows the results of a meta-analysis of 20 case-control studies of familial colorectal cancer risk undertaken by Johns and Houlston in 2001. The figures given in this table are relative risks compared to the general population risk, which in the Western world is approximately 1 in 20. Factors observed to contribute a greater risk were early age of onset, having two or more affected relatives, and a family history of

Table 8.10. (See Example 4).

Probability	Heterozygous	Not Heterozygous
Prior	0.5	0.5
Conditional		
No polyps at age 20 years	0.2	1
Joint	0.1	0.5

Posterior probability that consultand is heterozygous for FAP equals
$0.1/(0.1 + 0.5) = 1/6$

FAP, familial adenomatous polyposis.

Table 8.11. Empiric Relative Risks for Familial Colorectal Cancer

Type of Cancer	One Affected First-Degree Relative	Two or More First-Degree Relatives
Colorectal	2.25	4.25
Colon	2.42	5.81
Rectal	1.89	2.34

Source: Adapted from Johns and Houlston (2001).

Table 8.12. Family History Criteria for Triaging into High-, Moderate-, and Low-Risk Groups (UK Eastern Region Policy for Family History of Bowel Cancer 2000)

High Risk

Families with, or a good probability of, a hereditary CRC syndrome, either one of the polyposes, e.g. FAP, AFAP, PJS, or familial JPS, or HNPCC.

Moderate Risk

"Moderate risk" can be split into "high moderately increased risk" and "low–moderately increased risk" subgroups as defined below with each subgroup warranting somewhat different surveillance. Note that the criteria for "low–moderately increased risk" are exclusive, and any relevant family history over and above them will categorize the family as "high–moderately increased risk"

Low–Moderately Increased Risk

Two CRC-affected FDR with average age >60 years
One CRC-affected FDR and one CRC/HRC-affected SDR (both on the same side of the family) both < 70 years old

High–Moderately Increased Risk

For example, but not exclusively:
One CRC-affected FDR (45 years but > 35 years (if < 35 years, then > 50% chance of HNPCC, i.e., "high risk")
Two CRC-affected FDR with average age < 60 years (including both parents)
Two CRC-affected FDR and one CRC/HRC-affected FDR or SDR (but AC2-negative)
One CRC-affected FDR and two CRC/HRC-affected FDR or SDR (but AC2-negative)
NB. These are only common examples of 'high–moderately increased risk' and this list is not exhaustive. Clinical judgement will be required in situations where the family history is more than "high–moderately increased risk," but does not satisfy high risk/HNPCC criteria.

Low Risk

One CRC-affected FDR aged > 45 years and no CRC/HRC-affected SDR
No affected FDR and only one or two affected SDR

CRC, colorectal cancer, FAP, familial adenomatous polyposis; AFAP, attenuated FAP; PJS, Peutz-Jeghers syndrome; JPS, juvenile polyposis; HNPCC, hereditary nonpolyposis CRC; FDR, first-degree relative; SDR, second-degree relative; HRC, HNPCC related cancer; AC2, Amsterdam Criteria 2.

Source: Reproduced from Firth and Hurst (2005).

colon as opposed to rectal cancer. When analyzed by age at diagnosis in the affected individual, the relative risks with one affected relative were 3.87, 2.25, and 1.89 for ages <45 years, 45–59 years, and >59 years, respectively. The pooled relative risk for siblings (2.57) was significantly greater than that for offspring (2.26).

Categorization into high-moderate, moderate–low, and low risk based on the family history is somewhat arbitrary. One approach is summarized in Table 8.12. Screening and surveillance are tailored according to the category in which an individual falls. Those who fall in the high-moderate risk group are offered colonoscopy every 5 years commencing at age 45 years, or 5 years below the earliest age of onset in the family if that is lower. Those in the moderate-low category are offered a single one-time colonoscopy at age 55 years with follow-up colonoscopy 3 years later if an adenoma is identified. Those in the low-risk category are reassured and offered advice on lifestyle factors such as diet and exercise.

Key Point 2

The approach to risk assessment for individuals with a family history of colorectal cancer is similar to that for individuals with a family history of breast cancer. It is particularly important to identify a family history that would be consistent with a single-gene diagnosis such as FAP or HNPCC. These account for 2%–3% of all cases of colorectal cancer. Other genetic factors, which convey a lower risk, are involved in around 10%–20% of cases. Individuals with a family history of colorectal cancer can be counseled using epidemiological data and classified into high-moderate, moderate-low and low risk categories, depending upon the family's pattern of involvement.

Further Reading

Eeles, R.A., Easton, D.F., Ponder, B.A.J., and Eng, C. (eds.). (2004). *Genetic predisposition to cancer*, 2nd ed. Arnold, London.

Hodgson, S.V. and Maher, E.R. (1999). *A practical guide to human cancer genetics*, 2nd ed. Cambridge University Press, Cambridge.

Morrison, P.J., Hodgson, S.V., and Haites, N.E. (2002). Familial breast and ovarian cancer. Cambridge University Press, Cambridge.

Offit, K. (1998). *Clinical cancer genetics: Risk counseling and management.* Wiley-Liss, New York.

9

Balanced Chromosome Rearrangements

Balanced chromosome rearrangements are those in which there is no overall loss or gain of chromosome material. Unlike single-gene disorders, for which precise calculation of risks to offspring is usually possible, the segregation of chromosome rearrangements does not readily conform to any mathematical model that permits exact risk figures to be derived. Therefore, the genetic counselor faces a difficult task when presented with an individual known to carry a balanced chromosome rearrangement. To some extent, this role is eased by the widespread availability of prenatal diagnostic cytogenetic services, so that the provision of a precise risk for malsegregation might be viewed as being of minor importance and very much subsidiary to a discussion of the hazards and limitations of invasive prenatal diagnosis. Nevertheless, many individuals, particularly those for whom selective termination of pregnancy is unacceptable, will wish to know the likelihood that a pregnancy could result in an abnormal baby, and it could reasonably be argued that it is a dereliction of duty for a genetic counselor not to undertake risk assessment on an individual basis. Those with a special interest in this field are advised to refer to the excellent monograph entitled *Chromosome Abnormalities and Genetic Counseling* by Gardner and Sutherland (2004).

The difficulties posed by the lack of a simple mathematical method for predicting how a balanced rearrangement will segregate have been resolved at least in part by the increasing availability of empiric data derived from large collaborative studies. In some situations, these data allow very precise risk information to be given with confidence. For example, reliable risk figures are now available for all of the commonly encountered Robertsonian translocations, as outlined in Section 9.2. Unfortunately, specific empiric data are not usually available for reciprocal translocations, most of which are unique to the family in which they are encountered. However, by drawing on the information provided by large multicenter studies, it is often possible to arrive at a reasonable risk estimate for an individual family, and it is with this particular approach that this chapter is primarily concerned. Note that throughout this chapter, attention is paid primarily to the risk for viable imbalance, i.e., a surviving handicapped baby, rather than spontaneous miscarriage or infertility, since it is the possibility of having an abnormal child that tends to be of greatest concern to most prospective parents referred to a genetics clinic.

Risk and Mode of Ascertainment

Balanced chromosome rearrangements can be ascertained in many ways, and in turn can be associated with quite different reproductive outcomes. For example, ascertainment can be through an abnormal liveborn infant, a malformed stillborn infant, recurrent miscarriage, or infertility. Ascertainment can also occur purely by chance, as for example when an inherited balanced rearrangement is identified at a prenatal diagnosis carried out primarily to exclude Down syndrome. It is predictable that a relationship exists between the mode of ascertainment and the risk that malsegregation will lead to viable imbalance. (*Malsegregation* refers to meiotic segregation resulting in a gamete with an unbalanced chromosome complement.) If, for example, a balanced parental rearrangement has been identified following the delivery of an abnormal baby, then clearly this rearrangement has proved its potential for generating viable imbalance. It is likely that such a rearrangement will convey a higher risk for viable imbalance than one ascertained through investigations for recurrent miscarriage or infertility. In general, this holds true, but it is important to remember that there is no direct causal relationship between mode of ascertainment and risk. In other words, it would be wrong to base a risk purely on how a rearrangement has been ascertained. Instead, each rearrangement should be evaluated on an individual basis with a careful assessment of, first, the degree of imbalance that could be generated by malsegregation and, second, whether or not this could be associated with viability. The fallacy of basing risk prediction solely on the mode of ascertainment is amply illustrated by considering a family in which the same rearrangement has caused recurrent miscarriage in one member and the birth of an abnormal baby in other members. It would be illogical to quote different risks to different family members.

Interchromosomal Effect

Another issue that has clouded genetic counseling for balanced chromosome rearrangements is that of a possible *interchromosomal effect*. This refers to the possibility that a balanced rearrangement might somehow interfere with the meiotic process, resulting in the generation of a different and apparently unrelated chromosome abnormality. Concern about a possible interchromosomal effect has usually stemmed from the retrospective discovery that the parent of a newborn baby with an abnormality such as trisomy has a balanced rearrangement such as an inversion or a translocation. Detailed analyses, together with sperm chromosome studies in males with balanced rearrangements, have not provided support for an interchromosomal effect, with the possible exception of a recent report of an increased incidence of nontranslocation related aneuploidy in in vitro fertilization (IVF) embryos of fathers with Robertsonian translocations (Gianaroli et al., 2002). However, natural selective pressures appear to minimize this effect in term deliveries. Thus, at present, there is little if any justification for predicting an increased risk of chromosome abnormalities other than those directly related to the balanced parental rearrangement.

9.1 Reciprocal Translocations

A reciprocal translocation is formed when a break occurs in each of two chromosomes and the segments are exchanged to form two new "derivative" chromosomes. If no loss or gain of chromosome material occurs, the arrangement is described as *balanced*. A Robertsonian translocation is a particular type of reciprocal translocation in which the breakpoints are situated at or close to the centromeres of two acrocentric chromosomes. Robertsonian translocations are considered in Section 9.2.

Balanced reciprocal translocations involving two autosomes are relatively common, with an estimated incidence of approximately 1 in 500. Consequently, they constitute a significant proportion of all chromosome-related referrals to genetics clinics. Formerly, it was customary to quote an average risk of around 5%–10% for viable imbalance, and often a risk estimate of this nature will be appropriate. However, in some instances the risk will be much higher and in others it will be negligible. It is therefore essential that an attempt be made to assess each translocation on an individual basis. Details of how this can be undertaken will now be considered.

Segregation of a Reciprocal Translocation

It is likely that many factors are involved in determining how a particular reciprocal translocation will segregate. These include the relative lengths of the chromosomes and chromosome segments involved, the position of the centromeres, the position and frequency of chiasmata formation, and, perhaps primarily, the geometrical shape of the structure formed in meiosis I, when the homologous chromosomes involved in the translocation try to pair. In assessing the probable chromosome content of segregating gametes, it is customary to proceed on the basis that pairing of homologous chromosomes at meiosis I will be complete. In the case of a reciprocal translocation, this will involve the formation of a quadrivalent.

An example of a reciprocal translocation, along with its meiotic quadrivalent, is illustrated in Figure 9.1. The shape of the quadrivalent depends on the lengths of the translocated segments (t) and the "host" centric segments (c). Table 9.1 lists the most common ways in which the centromeres of a quadrivalent separate during meiosis I. All gametes generated by alternate segregation result in phenotypically normal offspring, with either normal chromosomes or the balanced rearrangement. In adjacent-1 segregation, adjacent nonhomologous centromeres cosegregate so that all gametes are unbalanced, being nullisomic for one translocated segment and disomic for the other. In adjacent-2 segregation, adjacent homologous centromeres cosegregate so that, once again, all gametes are unbalanced, in this instance being nullisomic for one centric

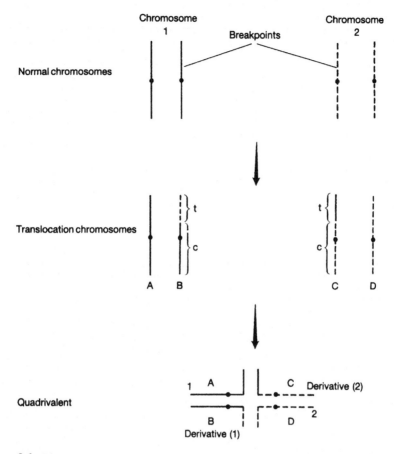

Figure 9.1. The generation of a balanced reciprocal translocation between chromosomes 1 and 2, with formation of a quadrivalent in meiosis: t = translocated segment, c = centric segment. See Table 9.1 for an explanation of meiotic segregation of this quadrivalent.

segment and disomic for the other. In most translocations the centric segment is larger than the translocated segment, so that adjacent-2 segregation is usually associated with much greater imbalance than adjacent-1 segregation. In addition, 3:1 segregation will lead to all gametes being unbalanced, with either 24 or 22 chromosomes, and the zygote having either 47 or 45 chromosomes. Thus, this results in either trisomy or monosomy for one of the nontranslocation chromosomes (interchange) or for one of the derivative chromosomes (tertiary).

Practical Approach to Risk Estimation

In the absence of full understanding of the mechanisms underlying segregation of a reciprocal translocation, the ideal approach for counseling would be the use of empiric data obtained from careful study and analysis of several families in

Table 9.1. Segregation of a Reciprocal Translocation

Pattern of Segregation	Gamete Chromosomes	Outcome of Zygote
2:2		
Alternate	A + D	Normal
	B + C	Balanced
Adjacent-1	A + C	Trisomy 1t Monosomy 2t
	B + D	Monosomy 1t Trisomy 2t
Adjacent-2	A + B	Trisomy 1c Monosomy 2c
	C + D	Monosomy 1c Trisomy 2c
3:1		
Trisomy	A + B + C	Trisomy 1 (interchange)
	A + B + D	Trisomy 1c2t (tertiary)
	A + C + D	Trisomy 1t2c (tertiary)
	B + C + D	Trisomy 2 (interchange)
Monosomy	A	Monosomy 2 (interchange)
	B	Monosomy 1t2c (tertiary)
	C	Monosomy 1c2t (tertiary)
	D	Monosomy 1 (interchange)

The segregation of a reciprocal translocation based on the example shown in Figure 9.1. t, translocated segment; c, centric segment.

which the specific translocation in question has been detected. Unfortunately, with very few exceptions, most reciprocal translocations are individually rare, if not unique, so that the limited empiric data available regarding mode of segregation have usually been obtained by pooling information from large numbers of families with different rearrangements. Studies of this nature have shown that viable imbalance in newborn babies results from adjacent-1 segregation in approximately 70%, 3 to 1 segregation in 25%, and adjacent-2 segregation in 5% of all cases (Cohen et al., 1994). It must be stressed that these figures represent pooled data and should not be used for counseling purposes. The translocation (11;22) (q23.3;q11.2) is unusual in that it is relatively common and is considered separately at the end of this section.

If the family concerned is very large and has been extensively investigated, it may be possible to derive an empiric recurrence risk through careful analysis of the extended pedigree. In segregation analysis of this nature, great care must be taken to identify all probands and exclude them from the calculation, so that in practice the limited size of most families will mean that it is usually impossible to derive a satisfactory risk. An example of how analysis can be undertaken in a large family is given below.

Figure 9.2 shows the pedigree of an extended kindred ascertained through the birth of an infant with an unbalanced karyotype. This is the proband, as indicated with a single arrow. The key point in the derivation of risks is to ensure that any individual in the pedigree whose existence has prompted chromosome studies in a further generation or sibship is classified as a secondary proband and excluded from the analysis. Essentially this means that both the proband and his/her immediate antecedents (i.e., the secondary probands) are not included in the risk calculation.

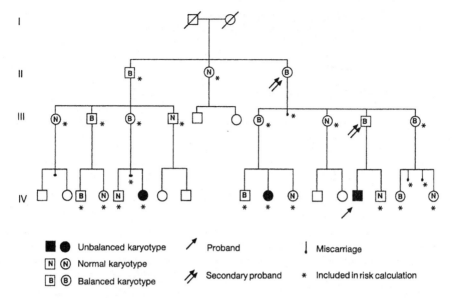

	Unbalanced karyotype	/ Proband	↓ Miscarriage
	Normal karyotype		
	Balanced karyotype	// Secondary proband	* Included in risk calculation

Figure 9.2. Pedigree of a large family in which a balanced reciprocal translocation is segregating. See Table 9.2.

From Figure 9.2 a table can be constructed showing the offspring of individuals with balanced chromosomes in each generation (Table 9.2). In this table it can be seen that 2 out of 23 offspring have an unbalanced viable karyotype, i.e., a risk of approximately 9%.

As a compromise between the use of pooled data, which are inappropriate, and complete understanding of segregation, which has yet to be achieved, the following approach has proved to be reasonably robust (Barisic et al., 1996; Midro et al., 1992). This involves four basic steps:

1. Identification of the breakpoints
2. Determination of which pattern(s) of malsegregation will give the smallest imbalance

Table 9.2. Derivation of Risks from Figure 9.2

Generation	Normal Karyotype	Balanced Karyotype	Unbalanced Karyotype	Miscarriage
II	1	1		
III	3	4		1
IV	5	3	2	3
Total	9	8	2	4

3. Assessment of viability of this imbalance
4. Estimation of overall risk for viability

1. The Breakpoints

These can usually be obtained from the cytogenetics report, which might read as follows: 46, XY,t(2;4)(p23;q31). This would indicate that breakage and subsequent reunion have occurred at band 23 on the short arm (p) of chromosome 2 and band 31 on the long arm (q) of chromosome 4.

2. Segregation Giving the Smallest Imbalance

Jalbert et al. (1980) have proposed that this can be assessed most easily by construction of a *pachytene diagram* (Fig. 9.3). This is obtained by drawing out the quadrivalent that would be seen in the pachytene stage of meiosis I, assuming that the homologous chromosomes involved in the translocation show complete pairing. The pachytene diagram is constructed taking into account the exact lengths of the chromosomes involved, using the data provided in Appendix A3.

The segregation producing the smallest imbalance can usually be identified by drawing a line between the homologous segments of the two longest arms of the quadrivalent. In general, adjacent-1 segregation gives rise to the smallest imbalance when the translocated segments are shorter than the centric segments, whereas adjacent-2 segregation generates the smallest imbalance when the opposite applies. There are a few important exceptions to these generalizations when, for example, the short arms of acrocentric chromosomes are involved, since imbalance of these has no obvious clinical effect.

Three-to-one segregation tends to yield the smallest degree of imbalance when one of the derivative chromosomes is very small or when the translocation involves chromosome 13, 18, or 21. Viable imbalance usually results from tertiary trisomy, although a few live-born infants with tertiary monosomy have been reported. Interchange trisomy is generally viable for only chromosomes 13, 18, and 21. Interchange monosomy is not viable for any of the autosomes. It is notable that 3:1 segregation resulting in abnormal live-born offspring occurs more often in female than in male carriers. This is in contrast to both adjacent-1 and adjacent-2 segregation, in which male and female carriers show roughly equal risks for generating viable imbalance.

Finally, it is very important to note that a few translocations have been observed to produce abnormal live-born infants by different modes of malsegregation, so that every pachytene diagram should be examined carefully to determine whether a relatively small degree of imbalance could be generated by more than one pattern of malsegregation.

3. Viability of the Imbalance

Having established which pattern(s) of malsegregation is likely to result in the smallest degree of imbalance, the next step is to try to determine whether this imbalance could be compatible with survival, i.e., viable. This can be done in two ways.

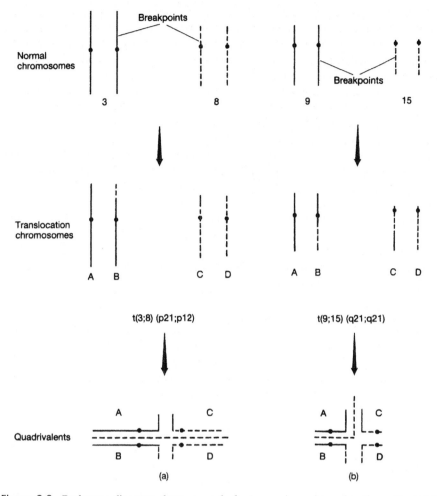

Figure 9.3. Pachytene diagrams drawn to scale for two reciprocal translocations. The bold dashed line indicates the pattern of segregation that will produce the smallest imbalance. In (a) this will be adjacent-1 segregation and in (b) 3:1 segregation resulting in interchange monosomy or trisomy.

The first, and more reliable, method involves review of contemporary information resources to see if the particular imbalance has ever been documented. This can be achieved most readily by reference to one of the standard textbooks of chromosome abnormalities (e.g., Schinzel, 2001), or to a computerized database (Schinzel, 1994), or to one of the databases now maintained online (e.g., the European Cytogeneticists Association Register of Unbalanced Chromosome Aberrations at www.ecaruca.net, or "Unique" at www.rare.chromo.org). If it is likely that the smallest imbalance will be generated by adjacent-1 segregation resulting in partial trisomy/monosomy, then it is essential to establish whether one or both of these imbalances has ever been observed. If neither has been described, then the risk for viability can safely be assumed to be extremely low. If only one has been described, then once again, the risk will be very low. In general, a combination of trisomy and monosomy is much less viable than either acting individually. It should be remembered that the viability of both trisomy/monosomy combinations should be assessed. For the translocation shown in Figure 9.1, this would involve assessment of trisomy 1p with monosomy 2p followed by trisomy 2p with monosomy 1p.

If this approach is unhelpful, then measurement of the extent of the imbalance can be used. This is not ideal, as it is apparent that viability of chromosome imbalance is not necessarily directly proportional to the length of the autosomal segments involved. For example, trisomy 13 is viable, albeit usually with early lethality in infancy, whereas trisomy 16 is incompatible with survival beyond early pregnancy. Nevertheless, support for a relationship between length of chromosome imbalance and viability is provided by evidence that observed neonatal aneuploidy lies to the left of a line joining 4% trisomy to 2% monosmy in 95% of published cases (Cohen et al., 1994; Daniel, 1979) (see Fig. 9.4). Thus, a table of chromosome segment size can be used (Daniel, 1985) (see Appendix 3) to determine the degree of imbalance and whether it falls within these limits.

4. Overall risk for Viable Imbalance

If careful appraisal of the pachytene diagram and/or the family history indicates that one or more malsegregation outcomes could be viable, then it is clearly desirable to try to estimate the overall probability that a pregnancy will result in an abnormal live-born infant. This will depend on the probability of malsegregation and the

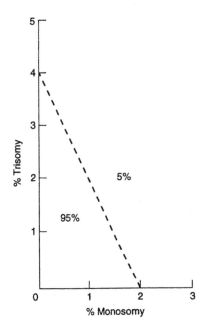

Figure 9.4. Most published cases (95%) of viable autosomal imbalance fall within the triangle defined by 4% trisomy and 2% monosomy. (Cohen et al., 1994; Daniel, 1979.)

likelihood of subsequent viability. Unfortunately, there is no reliable way in which the probability of malsegregation can be predicted. Reviews of the chromosome complements in sperm of men carrying a reciprocal translocation indicate that, on average, the percentages of alternate, adjacent-1, adjacent-2, and 3-1 segregation are approximately 40%–45%, 26%–36%, 12%–13%, and 5%–15%, respectively, but these figures show quite marked variation for different rearrangements (Benet et al., 2005). In addition, these figures do not correlate with estimates of subsequent viability, so that in practice this information cannot be used to facilitate risk prediction, although these data provide a useful starting point when estimating the likelihood that an abnormal sperm could be selected by a technique such as intracytoplasmic sperm injection (ICSI) in assisted conception. The very high proportions of abnormal sperm identified in most male translocation carriers clearly justify preimplantation diagnosis.

If the family concerned is sufficiently large to enable a "private" recurrence risk to be derived, then this is obviously the desirable course of action, remembering that the 95% confidence limits will be wide for a risk derived using small numbers. If the family is not sufficiently large to enable a private recurrence risk to be derived, then empiric data can be used. If one of the breakpoints has occurred in a terminal or acrocentric short arm region so that the risk of imbalance will be for a single segment (pure trisomy or monosomy), then it is possible to use very extensive information provided by analysis of over 1000 pedigrees (Stengel-Rutkowski et al., 1988) (see Table 9.3). For reciprocal translocations specifically involving the short arm of chromosome 4, the risk for viable single-segment imbalance varies from 47% for translocations with a breakpoint in 4p16 or 4p15 to 17% if the breakpoint is in 4p14 and 7% if the breakpoint lies in or between 4p13 and the centromere (Stengel-Rutkowski et al., 1984).

For reciprocal translocations predisposing to double-segment imbalance (i.e., duplication with deletion = partial monosomy/trisomy), empiric data from large numbers of families in which an identical translocation is segregating are not readily available with the exception of the 11q; 22q translocation, which is discussed below. In these difficult and relatively common situations, Stene and Stengel-Rutkowski (1988) have suggested that an estimate of the risk for viable imbalance can be made by determining the risk for each single-segment imbalance (Table 9.3) and then halving the lower value. An alternative resource is the website maintained by the Joseph Fourier University in Grenoble (http://hcforum.imag.fr), which derives risks for viable imbalance based on a rather complex logistic regression model (Cans et al., 1993). After inserting details of the translocation with the precise breakpoints, this facility provides an illustration of the pachytene diagram, together with details of potentially viable patterns of malsegregation and an indication of the overall risk for viable imbalance, depending upon the sex of the transmitting parent. (Generally, the sex of the transmitting parent is relevant only when 3:1 malsegregation could result in viable imbalance.)

For reciprocal translocations predisposing to 3:1 segregation, the risks for viable tertiary trisomy in offspring are usually less than 3% and 1% for female and male carriers, respectively (Stengel-Rutkowski et al., 1988). It is particularly important to consider this possibility when one of the derivative translocation chromosomes

Table 9.3. Risks for Unbalanced Live-Born Offspring When Imbalance Involves Only a Single Segment

Chromosome	Short Arm Band/Segment	Risk for Viable Imbalance	Long Arm Band/Segment	Risk for Viable Imbalance
1	34–11	$\dfrac{0}{21}$	43–42	$\dfrac{6}{49}$ (12.24%)
			32–23	$\dfrac{0}{39}$
			22–12	$\dfrac{0}{33}$
2	23–21	$\dfrac{2}{35}$ (5.71%)	35–33	$\dfrac{8}{35}$ (22.86%)
	16–13	$\dfrac{0}{20}$	32–31	$\dfrac{0}{30}$
	12–11	$\dfrac{0}{7}$	23–11	$\dfrac{0}{13}$
3	25–22	$\dfrac{2}{7}$ (28.57%)	ter–21	$\dfrac{0}{44}$
	21	$\dfrac{0}{22}$	13–12	$\dfrac{0}{4}$
	14–11	$\dfrac{0}{12}$		
4	16–14	$\dfrac{16}{80}$ (20%)	ter–21	$\dfrac{1}{128}$ (0.78%)
	13–11	$\dfrac{2}{27}$ (7.41%)		
5	14	$\dfrac{5}{17}$ (29.41%)	35–34	$\dfrac{9}{36}$ (25%)
	13	$\dfrac{7}{100}$ (7%)	33–31	$\dfrac{1}{13}$ (7.69%)
	12–11	$\dfrac{2}{61}$ (3.28%)		
6	ter–21	$\dfrac{1}{76}$ (1.32%)	26–21	$\dfrac{4}{14}$ (28.57%)
			16–11	$\dfrac{0}{8}$
7	21–15	$\dfrac{4}{21}$ (19.05%)	ter–22	$\dfrac{0}{63}$
	13–11	$\dfrac{2}{46}$ (4.35%)		
8	23–11	$\dfrac{6}{66}$ (9.09%)	24–21	$\dfrac{3}{27}$ (11.11%)
			13–12	$\dfrac{1}{49}$ (2.04%)
9	23–21	$\dfrac{9}{56}$ (16.07%)	ter–21	$\dfrac{0}{60}$
	13–11	$\dfrac{3}{47}$ (6.38%)	13–11	$\dfrac{0}{41}$

Table 9.3. (*continued*)

Chromosome	Short Arm Band/Segment	Risk for Viable Imbalance	Long Arm Band/Segment	Risk for Viable Imbalance
10	13–12	$\frac{3}{16}$ (18.75%)	25	$\frac{7}{50}$ (14%)
	11	$\frac{3}{64}$ (4.69%)	24	$\frac{5}{85}$ (5.88%)
			23–22	$\frac{0}{35}$
11	13–11	$\frac{0}{13}$	23	$\frac{3}{43}$ (6.98%)
			22–13	$\frac{0}{19}$
12	11	$\frac{3}{32}$ (9.36%)	ter–21	$\frac{0}{33}$
13			ter–11	$\frac{2}{128}$ (1.55%)
14			ter–11	$\frac{1}{99}$ (1.01%)
15			ter–21	$\frac{1}{37}$ (2.7%)
16	11	$\frac{5}{60}$ (8.33%)	ter–11	$\frac{0}{19}$
17	ter–11	$\frac{0}{18}$	23–21	$\frac{2}{20}$ (10%)
			12–11	$\frac{0}{4}$
18			22	$\frac{3}{20}$ (15%)
			21–11	$\frac{2}{75}$ (2.67%)
19			133	$\frac{3}{27}$ (11.11%)
			11	$\frac{0}{3}$
20	11	$\frac{5}{25}$ (20%)	ter–11	$\frac{0}{17}$
21			22–21	$\frac{4}{29}$ (13.79%)
22			ter–11	$\frac{0}{19}$

Source: Adapted from Tables 6a–d in Stengel-Rutkowski et at. (1988) with permission.

is very small and contains chromosome segments that are both viable as single-segment imbalance.

The t(11;22)(q23;q11) Translocation

Most reciprocal translocations are rare, if not unique. However, reciprocal translocations involving the long arms of chromosomes 11 and 22 occur relatively commonly, to the extent that it has been possible to gather information about their segregation in large numbers of families. Only one type of unbalanced karyotype is ever observed in offspring of t(11;22)(q23;q11) carriers. This results from 3:1 malsegregation leading to tertiary trisomy for a small derivative number 22 chromosome. Segregation analysis of published cases has given an overall risk for viable imbalance of 2%, rising to 5% if malformed stillborn infants are included (Iselius et al., 1983). These figures were not influenced significantly by the sex of the carrier parent. Stene and Stengel-Rutkowski (1988) noted 9 abnormal cases among 241 pregnancies (3.7%) of female carriers, with no abnormal cases in the 77 pregnancies conceived by male carriers.

These relatively low figures contrast starkly with the very high proportions of sperm with unbalanced chromosome complements identified by FISH analysis of interphase sperm nuclei in male carriers of this translocation. Analysis of almost 4000 sperm from three such males showed that less than 30% had a normal or balanced chromosome complement, 14%–21% showed adjacent-1, 12%–31% showed adjacent-2, and 30%–40% showed 3:1 malsegregation (Benet et al., 2005). This striking illustration of natural selection pressure against unbalanced sperm and embryos emphasizes the importance of using data obtained from sperm chromosome studies when counseling prospective parents who are contemplating IVF using techniques such as ICSI.

Cryptic "Subtelomeric" Translocations

Reciprocal rearrangements with breakpoints very close to the telomeres represent a small but very important group of translocations, which can now be identified using commercially available sets of subtelomeric FISH probes. As the breakpoints are subtelomeric, the degree of imbalance resulting from random Mendelian segregation of bivalents, or adjacent-1 malsegregation from a quadrivalent, is extremely small, so that these arrangements generally convey very high risks for viable imbalance. In practice, the translocated segments are so minute that it is likely that the chromosomes pair as bivalents rather than quadrivalents. Thus, the predicted outcome in gametes would be normal—25%, balanced—25%, duplicated/deleted—25%, and deleted/duplicated—25%. If both unbalanced rearrangements are viable, the overall risk for viable imbalance will be close to 50%.

9.2 Robertsonian Translocations

A *Robertsonian translocation* is a particular form of reciprocal translocation in which the long arms of two acrocentric chromosomes [i.e., the D (13–15) and G

Key Point 1

Estimating risks for the offspring of translocation carriers is difficult, and each situation merits very careful assessment. Four key steps are necessary.

1. Precise identification of the breakpoints
2. Construction of a pachytene diagram to determine which mode(s) of segregation will give relatively small degrees of imbalance
3. Establishing whether this imbalance is likely to be viable
4. Estimation of the overall risk of malsegregation and subsequent viability

   When undertaking this exercise, several points should be kept in mind

1. In general, the more terminal the breakpoints, the smaller will be the degree of imbalance and the greater the risk for viable imbalance.
2. Single-segment imbalance, occurring when one of the breakpoints is in a terminal band or in the short arm of an acrocentric chromosome, tends to be more viable than double-segment imbalance.
3. The effects of monosomy are usually more severe than those of trisomy.
4. Reciprocal translocations ascertained through an abnormal live-born infant tend to be associated with a greater subsequent risk of viable imbalance than those ascertained during investigations for infertility or recurrent miscarriage. While this does not imply an absolute or causal relationship between mode of ascertainment and risk for viable imbalance, it is consistent with the axiom that if something has happened once, then it may happen again.
5. In adjacent-1 and adjacent-2 segregation, the sex of the carrier parent usually does not influence the risk for viable imbalance. In 3:1 segregation, risks for female carriers are usually higher than those for male carriers.

(21 and 22) groups] fuse at, or very close to, their centromeres. The short arms comprising multiple copies of genes coding for ribosomal RNA are lost, an event of no apparent clinical significance.

During pachytene in meiosis, homologous pairing of a Robertsonian translocation is achieved by the formation of a trivalent (Fig. 9.5). If alternate segregation occurs, then all gametes are potentially viable, i.e., those carrying A and C will have a normal chromosome complement, and those carrying B will have the balanced rearrangement. If adjacent segregation occurs, then all gametes will carry a chromosome imbalance, resulting either in trisomy or in monosomy. For example, a gamete inheriting A and B will be disomic for chromosome 13 and will thus result in trisomy 13 in the zygote. Alternatively, a gamete inheriting only A or C will be nullisomic for chromosome 21 or 13 and will result in monosomy 21 or 13 in the zygote.

For the acrocentric chromosomes, the only viable aneuploidies are trisomy 21 and trisomy 13. Thus, in general, the only Robertsonian translocations that convey a risk for viable imbalance are those involving chromosomes 13 and/or 21. Homologous balanced translocations involving either of these two chromosomes,

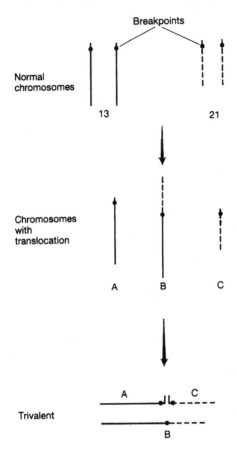

Figure 9.5. Shows the generation of a Robertsonian translocation involving chromosomes 13 and 21 and the formation of a trivalent in meiosis. Alternate segregation results in all gametes having either a normal (A and C) or balanced (B) chromosome complement. Adjacent segregation results in all gametes showing imbalance, either disomy (A and B or B and C) or nullisomy (A or C).

such as 45,XX,der(21;21)(q10;q10), will be associated with a risk of 100% for imbalance in all live-born offspring. Homologous Robertsonian translocations involving any of the other acrocentric chromosomes will be associated with a risk of 100% for either infertility or miscarriage. Note that a few carriers of a homologous Robertsonian translocation have produced live-born offspring as a result of monosomy or trisomy rescue, as discussed in the following section on uniparental disomy.

Recurrence Risks in Robertsonian Translocations

As with other reciprocal translocations, the likelihood that a carrier of a balanced Robertsonian translocation will have an abnormal baby relates to the probability of malsegregation and the subsequent viability of the chromosome imbalance. Chromosome studies on sperm from Robertsonian translocation carriers have shown that, on average, approximately 85% of sperm have a normal or balanced complement as a result of alternate segregation (Roux et al., 2005). Most of the remaining 15% have an unbalanced complement due to adjacent malsegregation. A small number of studies in female Robertsonian translocation carriers indicate that the proportion of unbalanced oocytes can exceed 30% (Munné et al., 2000). However, as with reciprocal translocations, there is strong selective pressure against conceptions with abnormal chromosomes, as revealed by the much lower frequencies of chromosome abnormalities seen in live-born infants born to Robertsonian translocation carriers.

Translocations Involving only D Group Chromosomes

In theory, both 13q14q and 13q15q translocations could result in the birth of infants with the clinical phenotype of Patau's syndrome (trisomy 13) due to adjacent malsegregation, but in practice this occurs very rarely. In a comprehensive review of published families in which a 13q14q translocation had been ascertained for various reasons, including four cases of Patau's syndrome, no other examples of malsegregation were detected among over 200 offspring of paternal and maternal carriers (Harris et al., 1979).

Similarly, in a large European collaborative prenatal study, there were no unbalanced offspring among 157 and 73 monitored pregnancies of female and male 13q14q carriers, respectively (Boué and Gallano, 1984). Nor were any unbalanced offspring detected in the pregnancies of 15 13q15q carriers. In a similar American collaborative prenatal study, there was 1 pregnancy with an unbalanced chromosome complement out of 86 from maternal 13q14q carriers and 1 out of 39 from paternal 13q14q carriers (Daniel et al., 1988).

Translocations Involving One D Group Chromosome and One Number 21 Chromosome

A painstaking analysis of 38 published families undertaken before banding permitted precise identification of individual chromosomes gave a risk of 10.1% ($\pm 1.8\%$) for a live-born infant with Down syndrome born to a female DqGq translocation carrier (Stene, 1970a). It was concluded that the risk for male carriers was much lower. All of these 38 families had been ascertained through a live-born infant with Down syndrome. The European collaborative prenatal study of 195 families, 174 of which were ascertained through a live-born infant with Down syndrome, gave recurrence risks for imbalance during the second trimester of 10% (2 out of 20) for 13q21q, 15.3% (21 out of 137) for 14q21q, and 11% (1 out of 9) for 15q21q translocations if the mother was the carrier (Boué and Gallano, 1984). No unbalanced karyotypes were diagnosed in pregnancies conceived by carrier fathers (0 out of 51 for 14q21q). Pooled data from the American collaborative prenatal study for 13q21q, 14q21q, and 15q21q carriers yielded a risk for Down syndrome of 12.7% (7 out of 55) for maternal carriers and 3.3% (1 out of 30) for paternal carriers (Daniel et al., 1988).

Thus, remembering that the prenatal figures are likely to overestimate the risk of imbalance at term, there is a clear consensus that the risk for live-born imbalance in offspring of 13q21q, 14q21q, and 15q21q female carriers is approximately 10%, with a much lower risk of around 1% for male carriers.

Translocations Involving One Number 21 Chromosome and One Number 22 Chromosome

The situation for 21q22q carriers is very similar to that outlined for Dq21q carriers. Analysis of seven families ascertained through a live-born infant with Down syndrome produced a risk estimate of 8.9% for female carriers (Stene, 1970b). The European collaborative prenatal study gave a risk for imbalance of 15.8% (3 out of 19) for maternal carriers, with no unbalanced offspring observed for paternal carriers (Boué and Gallano, 1984).

Uniparental Disomy and Robertsonian Translocations

Uniparental disomy (UPD) is the term used when both members of a pair of homologous chromosomes have been inherited from a single parent (see Section 10.6). In theory, a Robertsonian translocation could lead to UPD if adjacent segregation occurs yielding a disomic gamete, which is fertilized by a nullisomic gamete or by a monosomic gamete followed by jettisoning of the relevant homologue inherited from the noncarrier parent. This latter phenomenon is referred to as *trisomy rescue*. Alternatively, UPD could result from duplication of a single chromosome in a conceptus derived from a nullisomic gamete as a result of adjacent segregation (*monosomy rescue*). UPD becomes important only (1) if it doubles up a recessive allele or (2) if the relevant chromosome is imprinted. There is no evidence that chromosomes 13, 21, or 22 are imprinted, so that UPD for one of these chromosomes would not be expected to have any adverse phenotypic effect.

There is, however, clear evidence that both maternal and paternal UPD for chromosome 14 can result in phenotypic abnormalities (Kotzot and Utermann, 2005), and it is well recognized that maternal and paternal UPD for chromosome 15 results in the Prader-Willi and Angelman syndromes, respectively. There is therefore a theoretical possibility that carriers of a Robertsonian translocation involving either chromosome 14 or 15 could be at increased risk of having a child with a UPD syndrome. In practice, the risk appears to be low, with an observed overall incidence of 2 in 315 pregnancies (Silverstein et al., 2002). Although this risk is low, the severity of the clinical phenotype in the chromosome 15 UPD syndromes is such that

---

Key Point 2

Homologous Robertsonian translocations involving either or both number 13 or number 21 chromosomes will result in imbalance in all live-born offspring. Translocations involving one D group and one number 21 chromosome convey risks for Down syndrome in live-born offspring of maternal and paternal carriers of approximately 10% and 1%, respectively. Similar risks apply to the offspring of 21q22q carriers. The risk for Patau's syndrome in the live-born offspring of male and female 13q14q carriers is approximately 1%.

it is generally deemed appropriate to offer prenatal methylation or parent-of-origin studies whenever a translocation involving a number 15 chromosome is identified.

9.3 Three-Way Translocations

Three-way translocations involving reciprocal exchange between three autosomes are extremely rare, but on those infrequent occasions when a carrier presents at a genetics clinic, they constitute a major counseling problem. An example of a three-way translocation known to the author is shown in Figure 9.6. It was reported formally as 46,XX,t(3;12;5)(q24;q21.1;q11.1). This indicates that a segment of the

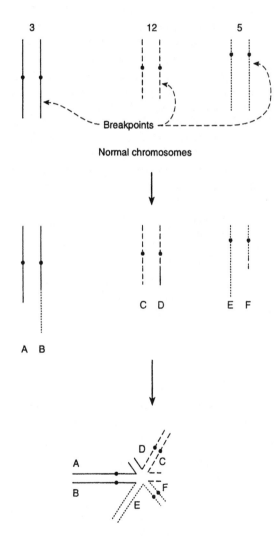

Figure 9.6. The generation of a balanced three-way reciprocal translocation involving chromosomes 3, 12, and 5, with subsequent formation of a hexavalent in meiosis. Alternate 3:3 segregation is the only mechanism that will result in a normal or balanced chromosome complement in a gamete.

long arm of one number 3 chromosome is present on the long arm of a number 12 chromosome. The segment from the long arm of number 12 is present on the long arm of one number 5 chromosome. The segment from the long arm of the number 5 chromosome is present on the long arm of the number 3 chromosome. As the woman in whom this rearrangement had been identified was entirely healthy, it was concluded that her three-way translocation was balanced. Ascertainment was because of recurrent pregnancy loss.

In order to predict the possible gamete chromosome complement, a multivalent diagram is constructed. This *hexavalent* permits homologous pairing of all six chromosomes. Alternate 3:3 segregation is the only pattern that will result in a normal or balanced chromosome constitution in the gamete, i.e., A + C + E will yield a normal chromosome constitution, and B + D + F will yield a balanced chromosome constitution. Other patterns of 3:3 segregation, such as adjacent-1 (nonhomologous centromeres, e.g., A, C, and F) or adjacent-2 (homologous centromeres, e.g., B, E, and F), will result in chromosome imbalance, which for all of the possible combinations will almost certainly not be viable. Similarly, 4:2, 5:1 and 6:0 segregation will all result in nonviable conceptions.

The approach to predicting the likelihood of viable imbalance is similar to that outlined for two-way reciprocal translocations in Section 9.1 in that, ideally, an attempt should be made to determine which patterns of segregation could occur and, by reference to suitable literature resources, to determine whether viability is possible. Sperm analysis in a male with a balanced 2,11,22 three-way translocation revealed that 87% had an abnormal chromosome complement (Cifuentes et al., 1998). This high incidence of sperm with unbalanced complements is reflected in empiric studies of pregnancy outcomes in three-way translocation carriers. Gorski et al. (1988) reviewed 25 literature reports of three-way translocations, most of which had been ascertained through the birth of an abnormal baby, and concluded that approximately 50% of recognized pregnancies ended in spontaneous miscarriage. Among the surviving pregnancies, roughly 80% were normal and 20% were abnormal. Batista et al. (1994) concluded on the basis of a literature review that the pattern of meiotic segregation resulting in viable imbalance is most frequently adjacent-1, followed by 4:2. They observed an overall risk for miscarriage of approximately 50%, with 26 out of 63 (41%) live-born infants having an unbalanced karyotype.

Key Point 3

Three-way translocations involving reciprocal exchange between autosomes are extremely rare. To assess offspring risks, a hexavalent should be drawn up to determine whether one or more patterns of segregation could result in viable imbalance. Empiric studies indicate that the risk of miscarriage is approximately 50% and that if viable imbalance is a possibility, the risk of an abnormal live-born infant is at least 20%.

9.4 Pericentric Inversions

A pericentric inversion is formed when two breaks occur on opposite arms of a chromosome with rotation of the intervening segment, this being a balanced rearrangement. Pericentric inversions probably constitute the most common rearrangements encountered in humans, with an estimated incidence of 1%–2%. Those involving only the heterochromatic regions close to the centromeres of chromosomes 1, 9, and 16 can be regarded as polymorphisms and are not associated with an increased risk of imbalance in progeny (Kaiser, 1984).

For other pericentric inversions there may well be a risk of viable imbalance in offspring. Once again, there is no precise mathematical model that allows this risk to be calculated. A logical approach has to involve consideration of the possible recombinants that could be generated by malsegregation at meiosis and subsequent viability of the resulting imbalance.

Segregation of a Pericentric Inversion

During meiosis a chromosome containing an inversion is likely to pair with its homologue, either by ballooning out of the inversion region if this is small or by formation of a loop that facilitates homologous pairing in bigger inversions (Fig. 9.7). If the inverted segment is very long, then it is likely that the inversion segments will pair directly, with nonpairing of the distal segments not involved in the rearrangement. If pairing of the inversion segments occurs, then a single or uneven number of crossovers occurring within the inverted segment will result in half of the chromatids receiving an unbalanced chromosome complement consisting of a combination of duplication of one distal noninverted segment with deficiency of the noninverted segment at the opposite end of the chromosome.

Since it is unlikely that imbalance will be viable if it exceeds more than 4%–5% of the haploid autosomal content (see Section 9.1), it is apparent that pericentric inversions will generally be associated with viable imbalance only if the inversion segment is long or, more specifically, if the noninverted segments are short. Thus, the probability that a balanced pericentric inversion will malsegregate to produce viable imbalance will depend on (1) the likelihood of a recombination in the inversion segment, and thus the size of the inversion segment, and (2) the viability of the resulting duplication/deficiency.

Sperm analysis in heterozygote pericentric inversion carriers has confirmed that there is a positive relationship between the likelihood of recombination and the size of the inverted segment, as measured in megabases (Mb) or expressed as a proportion of total chromosome length (Anton et al., 2005). For example, the proportion of recombinant gametes rises from zero when the size of the inversion is less than 50 Mb, to approximately 10% for 100 Mb inversions and to over 30% for inversions greater than 150 Mb. Similarly, the proportion of recombinant gametes is zero if the inversion is less than 25% of the total chromosome length and rises to 40% for inversions greater than 75% of the total chromosome length. Although the relationship between

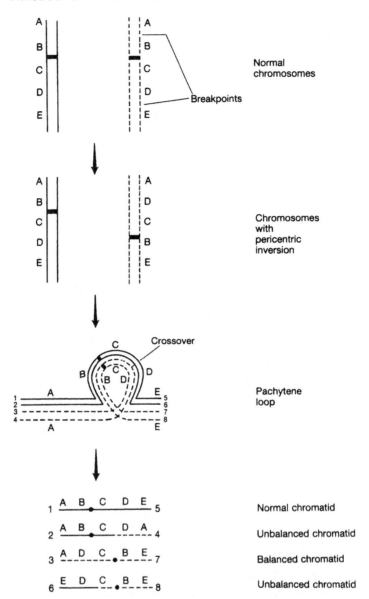

Figure 9.7. The generation of a pericentric inversion and loop formation in meiosis. If a single crossover occurs as indicated, then half of the chromatids will be unbalanced. Note that each chromosome is shown as consisting of two chromatids.

inversion size and frequency of recombination is not absolute, it is consistent with previous observations that the average segment size of inversions that have resulted in viable recombination is approximately 65% (measured as a proportion of the total chromosome length), with inversions of less than 30% of the chromosome size rarely resulting in the birth of an abnormal infant (Kaiser, 1984).

Practical Approach to Risk Estimation

This is very similar to the scheme outlined for reciprocal translocations and involves a four-step procedure as follows:

1. Identification of the breakpoints
2. Determination of the extent of imbalance that would be generated by an uneven number of crossovers if the inverted segment pairs with its normal homologue
3. Establishment of the potential viability of this imbalance
4. Estimation of the overall risk for viability

1. Identification of the Breakpoints

The report provided by an experienced cytogeneticist might be as follows: 46, XY,inv(2)(p21q37). This indicates that the breakpoints are at band 21 on the short arm (p) and band 37 on the long arm (q) of chromosome 2.

2. Extent of the Potential Imbalance

This can be deduced from the breakpoints. In the example above, recombination resulting in imbalance would produce either duplication (trisomy) for the distal portion of the short arm of chromosome 2 (pter to p21) with deletion (monosomy) for the distal portion of the long arm (q37 to qter), or vice versa.

3. Viability of the Imbalance

This can be assessed in several ways, as outlined for reciprocal translocations. The first involves reference to the literature (e.g., Schinzel's *Human Cytogenetics Database*, 1994, or Schinzel's *Catalogue*, 2001) to establish whether infants with either trisomy and/or monosomy for these segments have ever been reported. Another useful resource is the data provided by Ishii et al. (1997), who reviewed all reports of pericentric inversions published between 1981 and 1995 and presented details of those that had resulted in viable imbalance. Their data have been summarized in a concise table by Gardner and Sutherland (2004), which is reproduced here as Table 9.4.

Alternatively, careful measurement of the imbalance will indicate whether this falls within the observed 4%/2% limits of trisomy/monosomy found to be compatible with viability. Daniel (1981), who has pioneered and refined this approach, concluded that "the restrictions on the size of chromosome imbalance surviving until term are similar whether this imbalance arises from reciprocal translocations or pericentric inversions." In general, duplication (trisomy) is more viable than deletion (monosomy).

4. Overall Risk for Viability

This is the key question and, unfortunately, it cannot always be answered with certainty. However, a reasonable risk estimate can be made based on knowledge of

Table 9.4. Autosomal Pericentric Inversions Associated with
the Birth of a Recombinant Offspring

Chromosome	Inversions		
2	p25q35	p25.3q33.3	
3	p25q23	p25q25*	
4	p13q28	p15.32q35	
5	p13q33	p13q35	p14q35
	p15q32	p15.1q33.3	p15.1q35.1*
	p15.3q35		
6	p23q27	p23.07q25.13	
7	p14.2q36.3	p15q36	p15.1q36
	p22q22		
8	p23q22*	p23.3q24.1	
10	p11q26	p11.2q25.2*	p12q25
	p15q24		
11	p11q25	p13q23.3	
13	p11q21	p11q22	p12q13
	p12q14	p13q21*	p13q31
16	p13q22	p13.1q22	
17	p11q25	p13.3q25.1	
18	p11q11	p11.2q12.2	p11.2q21.3
20	p11.2q13.3	p12q13.3	p13q13.1
21	p11q21	p11.2q22.1	p12q22
22	p11q21	p13q12*	p13q12.2

*Reported in more than one family.

Source: Reproduced from Gardner and Sutherland (2004), with additional information kindly provided by the authors.

the extent of potential imbalance, method of ascertainment, and pooled empiric data. Ideally, it is desirable to try to derive a recurrence risk for each individual family based on analysis of the pedigree, but in practice this is not usually possible. Alternatively, figures have been derived for a few of the more common inversions associated with viable imbalance. For example, inversions with breakpoints at 13p12 and 13q21/22 convey a risk for viable imbalance of 7.25% in female carriers; the risk for male carriers is much lower (Pai et al., 1987). The risk for inversions with breakpoints at 18p11 and 18q11–22 is 8% (Ayukawa et al., 1994).

Sutherland et al. (1976) concluded, on the basis of a literature review, that if there was a previous viable recombinant in the family, then a risk of 5% for male and 10% for female inversion carriers would be "accurate enough for patients to arrive at informed decisions." A risk of 1% was suggested if there had been no viable recombinants in the family. Sherman et al. (1986) analyzed 216 pedigrees and obtained an overall recurrence risk for viable imbalance of 6.9% when ascertainment was through viable imbalance, compared with 1.2% when ascertainment was because of a balanced inversion. Once again, risks for female carriers tended to be higher than for male carriers. Sherman et al. also concluded that there was no significant deviation from the expected 1:1 segregation of balanced inversions to normal karyotypes among the offspring of both male and female carrier parents.

The results of the European (Boué and Gallano, 1984) and American (Daniel et al., 1988) collaborative prenatal studies are consistent with these observations. In the European study, 7 unbalanced fetal karyotypes were detected in 118 prenatal diagnoses (2 from 51 fathers, 5 from 67 mothers). Six of these unbalanced karyotypes occurred in families ascertained through previous viable imbalance, whereas only one unbalanced fetal karyotype was observed in 110 pregnancies ascertained for other reasons such as spontaneous miscarriage. In the American study, two recombinant karyotypes were detected in 102 pregnancies. One of these two recombinants occurred in a total of 11 pregnancies being monitored as a result of ascertainment through previous viable imbalance. Experience in France and Belgium confirms that most pericentric inversions convey a very low risk for viable malsegregation. In the French survey of 305 independent pericentric inversions, there were 8 cases of imbalance among 595 descendants of inversion carriers (Groupe de Cytogénéticiens Français, 1986a). The Belgian study reported a total of 2 unbalanced offspring, 1 of whom was a proband, amongst 57 live-born children of pericentric inversion carriers (Kleczkowska et al., 1987). Finally, an estimate of the risk for viable imbalance can be obtained from the website maintained by the Joseph Fourier University in Grenoble (http://hcforum.imag.fr). This deals with both pericentric and paracentric inversions, and provides details of which particular patterns of duplication/deficiency are likely to be viable together with a numerical estimate of the actual risk.

Key Point 4

The probability that a balanced pericentric inversion will result in viable imbalance is greatest when the inversion is long and the noninverted segments are short. As a practical approach to providing a risk for pericentric inversion carriers, it is appropriate to use the 5% and 10% figures quoted by Sutherland et al. (1976) if there is a history of previous viable imbalance in the family or if the imbalance generated by a crossover is likely to be viable as judged by length of imbalance and/or review of the literature. Otherwise, a figure of 1%–2% is a reasonable estimate of maximum risk.

9.5 Paracentric Inversions

A paracentric inversion is formed when two breaks occur in a single arm of a chromosome, with the intervening segment rotating to become inverted, this being a balanced rearrangement. The centromere is not involved, so the lengths of the chromosome arms are not altered. This may explain at least in part why paracentric inversions appear to be much less common than pericentric inversions, as without good banding, subtle paracentric inversions could easily go undetected.

Balanced paracentric inversions generally convey only a very low risk for viable imbalance in offspring. This can be explained by considering the outcome for short and long paracentric inversions. If the inversion is very small, then pairing in meiosis

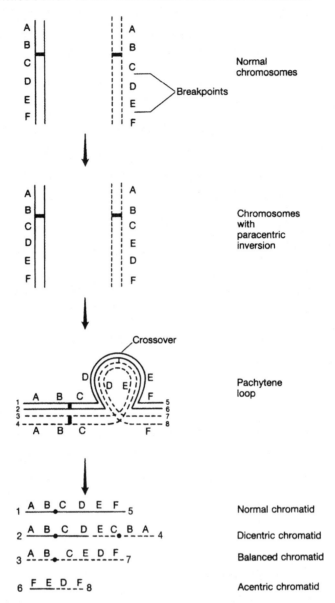

Figure 9.8. The generation of a paracentric inversion with loop formation in meiosis. All unbalanced chromatids generated by a crossover in the loop are likely to be unstable. Note that each chromosome is shown as consisting of two chromatids.

will probably proceed uneventfully. Alternatively, a small loop may be formed in pachytene (Fig. 9.8), and if no crossover occurs within the loop, then once again, all gametes will receive either the normal chromosome or the inverted chromosome with no risk of imbalance. Consequently, for very small paracentric inversions, in which crossing-over in the loop is unlikely, the risk for abnormal progeny will be very low. For larger paracentric inversions, there is a significant probability that recombination will occur within the pachytene loop between adjacent nonsister chromatids, although recent studies indicate that the proportion of recombinant gametes, even in carriers of relatively large inversions, is very low, usually less than 1% (Anton et al., 2005). As shown in Figure 9.8, if recombination occurs, half of the daughter chromatids will be unbalanced, being either acentric or dicentric. Consequently, there is considerable potential for the generation of unbalanced gametes, but almost invariably these will not be associated with viability, as acentric fragments are usually lost in an early mitotic division and dicentric chromosomes are inherently unstable due to their attachment to opposing spindle fibers.

Against this background, it is rather surprising that there has been a small number of reports of viable imbalance resulting from apparent malsegregation of a balanced paracentric inversion. In a review of over 400 cases, it was concluded that the incidence of viable recombinants was of the order of 3.8% (Pettenati et al., 1995). This high figure contrasted sharply with the much lower risks derived in other studies (Daniel et al., 1988; Groupe de Cytogénéticiens Français, 1986) and has been challenged on the basis of ascertainment bias and inclusion of many cases that were actually insertions rather than inversions (Madan and Nieuwint, 2002; Sutherland et al., 1995). The prevailing literature points to a consensus that it is generally reasonable to counsel on the basis that the risk is low, if not very low, i.e., less than 1%, but with the caveat that prenatal diagnostic surveillance should be available if requested.

Key Point 5

Small paracentric inversions are unlikely to result in unbalanced gametes, whereas any imbalance resulting from large paracentric inversions will usually be nonviable. Overall, the risk of viable imbalance in the offspring of a balanced paracentric inversion carrier is very low, although not negligible, so that the offer of prenatal monitoring would be a prudent precaution.

9.6 Insertions

These are rare balanced chromosome rearrangements that arise when two breaks occur in one chromosome, resulting in loss of the intervening segment, which becomes inserted into a different site on the same chromosome (intrachromosomal) or into a different chromosome (interchromosomal). Insertions are sometimes referred to as *insertional translocations*. Intrachromosomal insertions are also referred to as *shifts*.

Intrachromosomal Insertions

Intrachromosomal insertions can occur within an arm or between arms (Figs. 9.9 and 9.10). In both types, pairing at meiosis can be achieved by formation of two loops, with, for example, "ballooning out" of the inserted segment in the normal

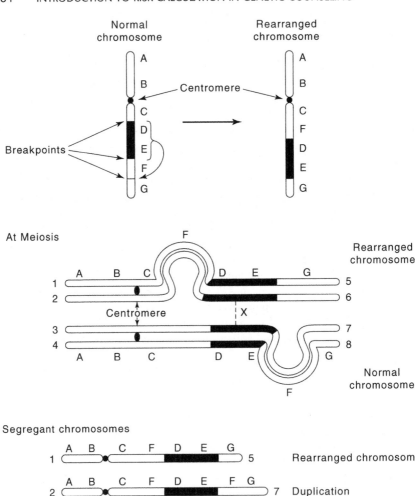

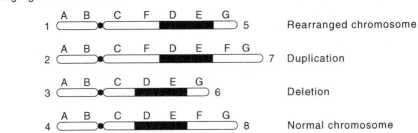

Figure 9.9. The generation of an intrachromosomal within-arm insertion and possible patterns of segregation at meiosis. X marks the site of a crossover. Note that at meiosis each chromosome is shown as consisting of two chromatids.

homologue at the site of its original position and in the derivative chromosome at the site of the insertion. A single or uneven number of crossovers between the ballooned-out segments will generate unbalanced recombinant chromosomes, so that if the segment between the two loops is large, a high incidence of gametes with an abnormal chromosome complement would be anticipated (Figs. 9.9 and 9.10).

Chromosome   Chromosome

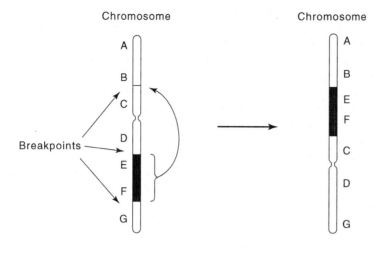

Breakpoints

At Meiosis

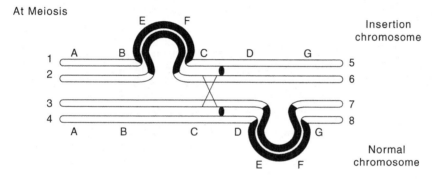

Insertion chromosome

Normal chromosome

Segregant chromosomes

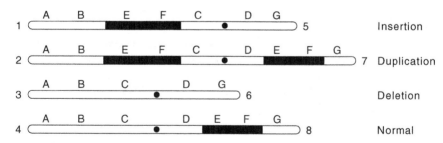

Figure 9.10. The generation of an intrachromosomal between-arm insertion and possible patterns of segregation at meiosis. X marks the site of a crossover. Note that at meiosis each chromosome is shown as consisting of two chromatids.

The observed risk of viable imbalance based on reviews of published cases is around 10%–15% (Madan and Menko, 1992; Vekemans and Morichon-Delvallez, 1990). In practice, each intrachromosomal insertion should be assessed on an individual basis. The risk is likely to be greater than 15% if the insertion is small, resulting in viable duplication or deletion, particularly if there is a long segment between the original site of the inserted segment and its new position, in which case it becomes more likely that a recombination event will occur. In these situations the theoretical risk for viable imbalance approaches 50%.

Interchromosomal Insertions

If an insertion involves two chromosomes, then a high risk of unbalanced gamete formation can be predicted, resulting either from random 2:2 segregation giving a risk of 50%, or from crossing-over in a loop in a quadrivalent formed by complete homologous pairing. In this latter situation, which is more likely to arise if the insertion segment is large, crossing-over will result in unbalanced gametes showing both duplication and deletion in contrast to random 2:2 segregation, which will result in either duplication or deletion but not both.

In practice, small interchromosomal insertions are associated with a high risk for viable imbalance. In the American prenatal collaborative study (Daniel et al., 1988), two of four offspring of balanced carriers were unbalanced. This study also reviewed four families previously reported in the literature with autosomal interchromosomal insertions and noted a risk of 41% (11 out of 27) for unbalanced full-term progeny, probands having been excluded. Doheny et al. (1997) noted a ratio of close to 1:1 for normal:abnormal live-born offspring among the offspring of female carriers. Van Hemel and Eussen (2000) collected data from 87 published cases and derived risks for an abnormal live-born infant of 32% and 36% for male and female carriers, respectively.

Key Point 6

Insertions convey a high risk for viable imbalance in the offspring of balanced carriers. For intrachromosomal insertions, the empiric pooled risk for viable imbalance is approximately 15%. In general, the smaller the size of the insertion, the greater the risk for viable imbalance. Interchromosomal insertions convey an even higher risk, approaching 50%, if duplication and/or deletion of the inserted segment are viable.

9.7 Rearrangements Involving an X Chromosome

X-Autosome Translocations

The consequences of balanced rearrangements involving an X chromosome are difficult to predict, both in terms of possible effects on the carriers and risks for imbalance in offspring. Balanced X-autosome translocations present a particularly difficult counseling problem. If X-chromosome inactivation occurs randomly in these women, then in approximately half of their cells the derivative X-autosome with an inactivation center is inactivated, resulting in a variable degree of functional autosomal monosomy with functional disomy for the translocated X-chromosome segment. This would be expected to have adverse phenotypic effects. In approximately 80% of women with a balanced X-autosome translocation, late replication and methylation studies show that the normal X chromosome is usually inactivated (Mattei et al., 1982; Schmidt and Du Sart, 1992). This explains why most females with a balanced X-autosome translocation are clinically normal and indicates that either X inactivation in the embryo occurs nonrandomly or that cell lines in which the normal X chromosome is randomly inactivated have a major selective advantage, as there is no loss of functional autosome activity.

Although around 80% of female carriers of a balanced X-autosome translocation are clinically normal, in approximately 50% of published cases they are infertile, and in these cases almost invariably one of the breakpoints is in the segment Xq13-26, which is believed to be a critical region for gonadal function (Therman et al., 1990). Almost all male carriers of an X-autosome translocation are infertile because of spermatogenic arrest attributable to disruption of the *sex vesicle*, this being the name given to the structure formed by the X and Y chromosomes when they pair at the pseudoautosomal regions in meiosis. When assessing risks for female carriers in which the X-chromosome breakpoint does not involve a critical region, it is appropriate to adopt the same strategy used when assessing risks for autosomal translocations, as outlined in Section 9.1. This involves constructing a diagram of the pachytene quadrivalent and then assessing which of the possible gamete chromosome complements could result in viable imbalance. This always requires detailed individual assessment, taking into account the possible effects of both autosomal and X-chromosome abnormalities (Schmidt and Du Sart, 1992). An added complication is that the effects of autosomal imbalance can be less severe than expected in a female if inactivation extends from the inactivation center on the derivative X chromosome to the translocated autosomal segment. In general, most fertile female carriers of a balanced X-autosome translocation run a relatively high risk for having a child with phenotypic abnormalities.

X-Chromosome Pericentric Inversions

Both male and female carriers of balanced pericentric X-chromosome inversions are generally entirely healthy, although if one of the breakpoints involves a critical region for ovarian function, then a female carrier could be infertile or develop premature menopause. Female carriers in whom the critical region is intact usually have entirely healthy surviving children, although a very small number of daughters with variable features of Turner's syndrome have been described (Schorderet et al., 1991). These features are a consequence of deletion and duplication resulting from recombination within an inversion loop. Loss of Xp is associated with short stature, whereas loss of Xq results in ovarian failure. A male embryo inheriting X-chromosome imbalance will almost certainly not be viable. Obviously, recombination cannot occur in an X chromosome in a male with a balanced pericentric inversion X, as most of the X chromosome does not pair with the Y chromosome. In these males, all daughters would be predicted to be healthy balanced carriers. Fertility in a male carrier of a balanced pericentric inversion X is usually not affected.

Key Point 7

Every rearrangement involving an X chromosome should be assessed on an individual basis, remembering that

1. most female carriers of a balanced X-autosome translocation are clinically normal.
2. almost all male carriers of a balanced X-autosome translocation are infertile.
3. any X chromosome breakpoint disrupting the "critical region" (Xq13-26) in a female is likely to result in infertility.
4. the possible effects in offspring of both autosomal monosomy/trisomy and X-chromosome nullisomy/disomy should be considered.

9.8 Case Scenario

Investigation of a 25-year-old man because of infertility and severe oligospermia showed that he carried a reciprocal translocation involving chromosomes 4 and 21. The formal cytogenetics report read as follows: 46,XY,t(4;21)(p14;q22.11). Since this man was otherwise healthy, it was concluded that his chromosome rearrangement was balanced. Subsequent investigations showed that his mother and sister also carried the rearrangement. There was no family history of recurrent miscarriage or malformed infants, and it was not possible to carry out chromosome analysis on other members of his mother's family.

When this man and his sister attended the genetics clinic, three specific questions arose:

1. Was this rearrangement the cause of the man's severe oligospermia?
2. If this man and his wife attempted to have a child using IVF and ICSI, what was the chance that a selected sperm would have an unbalanced chromosome complement?
3. What was the chance that his sister would have an abnormal baby?

In responding to the first question, it was pointed out that a small but significant proportion of men with an apparently balanced reciprocal translocation show infertility due to azospermia or severe oligospermia. In the absence of other possible explanations (bilateral absence of the vas deferens due to mild cystic fibrosis had been excluded), it was therefore likely that the translocation was responsible for his infertility. The full explanation for spermatogenic arrest in translocation carriers is not known, but it is thought to involve failure of complete pairing of homologous chromosomes in meiosis I, with disruption of the sex vesicle (the paired X and Y chromosomes), which is essential for successful spermatogenesis.

To answer the second question, reference was made to the relevant literature to establish whether sperm studies had ever been undertaken in another male with an identical or similar rearrangement. The review by Benet et al. (2005) lists 89 reciprocal translocations in which sperm studies have been undertaken. Unfortunately, none of these is between chromosomes 4 and 21. As a compromise, it was concluded that it was reasonable to quote the mean values derived by Benet et al., as outlined previously in this chapter in the section on reciprocal translocations (p. 167), i.e., less than 50% of sperm have a normal or balanced complement. Thus, this man was informed that the probability that a randomly selected sperm would have an unbalanced chromosome complement was slightly greater than 1 in 2. To date there does not appear to be any evidence that the chromosome content of a sperm influences its external appearance, so that a scientist cannot distinguish between "good" and "bad" sperm when making a selection for ICSI.

To try to determine the likelihood that this man's sister would have an abnormal live-born infant, a pachytene diagram was constructed (Fig. 9.11) and the various possible patterns of segregation were considered (Table 9.5). It was noted that this translocation with its relatively short translocated segments, comprising only 1.21% (4p14-4pter) and 0.445% (21q22.11-21qter) of the total genome, was particularly hazardous in that both adjacent-1 and 3:1 segregation could produce unbalanced oocytes, which, if fertilized, could result in abnormal live-born infants. Specifically, adjacent-1 segregation (B and D in Fig. 9.11) could result in a baby with both the

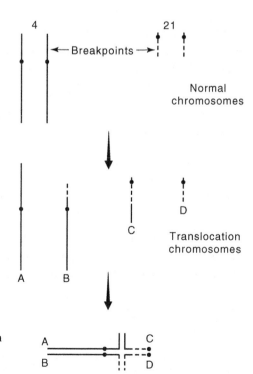

Figure 9.11. The pachytene diagram generated by a reciprocal translocation involving chromosomes 4 and 21. See the case scenario.

Table 9.5. Possible Segregation Patterns Resulting from a 4p14–21q22.11 Reciprocal Translocation (See Case Scenario and Figure 9.11)

Segregation	Chromosomes in Gamete	Outcome
Alternate	A and D	Normal karyotype
	B and C	Balanced karyotype
Adjacent-1	A and C	Trisomy 4pter-p14 and monosomy 21q22.11-qter. Probably viable.
	B and D	Monosomy 4pter-p14 and trisomy 21q22.11-qter. Probably viable.
Adjacent-2	A and B	Trisomy 4p14-qter and monosomy 21 pter-q22.11. Nonviable.
	C and D	Monosomy 4p14-qter and trisomy 21pter-q22.11. Nonviable.
3:1	A, C, and D	Tertiary trisomy 4pter-p14 and 21pter-q22.11. Possibly viable.
	B, C, and D	Interchange trisomy 21. Viable.
	A, B, and D	Tertiary trisomy 4p14-qter and 21q22.11-qter. Nonviable.
	A, B, and C	Interchange trisomy 4. Nonviable.
	A or B or C or D	Interchange or tertiary monosomy —all probably nonviable.

Wolf-Hirschhorn (4p-) syndrome and the partial phenotype of Down syndrome, as 21q22 harbors the so-called Down syndrome critical region. Adjacent-1 segregation could also result in an infant with trisomy for distal 4p and monosomy for distal 21q (A and C), and once again, this could be viable, as both have been reported in live-born infants. Three-to-one segregation could result in interchange trisomy 21 (B, C, and D), and it is just possible that tertiary trisomy for the derivative number 21 chromosome could also be viable (A, C, and D).

Having established that the translocation could malsegregate to cause viable imbalance, an attempt was made to quantify the risk. Stengel-Rutkowski et al. (1984) calculated that a breakpoint in 4p14 conveys a risk of 17% for viable single-segment imbalance, and as the chromosome 21 breakpoint is close to the telomere, it could be argued that this figure of 17% would be appropriate in this situation. Alternatively, reference to Table 9.3 yields risks for single-segment imbalance of 20% for 4p14 and 13.8% for 21q22 breakpoints. By adopting the suggestion of Stene and Stengel-Rutkowski (1988) that an estimate of total risk can be made by halving the lower of these two figures, an overall risk of 7% is obtained. To this we should probably add around 3%–5% to account for the possibility of 3:1 segregation and interchange trisomy 21. The man's sister was informed, therefore, that there was definitely a risk that she could have an abnormal baby because of the translocation, and that this risk was at least 10% and could be considerably higher.

This scenario emphasizes the importance of assessing each translocation on an individual basis and illustrates the difficulties encountered in reaching specific risk figures. For this translocation, the program available online at http://hcforum.imag.fr yielded risks of 21.1% (95% CI = 16.03%–27.27%) and 36.54% (95% CI = 30.87% –42.61%) for male and female carriers, respectively. Clearly, these risks are higher than those suggested here, and they may well be more appropriate. This makes the point that risk provision in these situations is an imprecise science, and that all possible approaches should be used to try to ensure that carriers of rearrangements are given an indication of the range of risks that can apply in each particular situation.

Further Reading

Borgaonkar, D.S. (1997). *Chromosomal variation in man*, 8th ed. John Wiley & Sons, New York.

Daniel, A. (ed.). (1988). *The cytogenetics of mammalian autosomal rearrangements*. A.R. Liss, New York.

Gardner, R.J.M. and Sutherland, G.R. (2004). *Chromosome abnormalities and genetic counseling*, 3rd ed. Oxford University Press, New York.

Schinzel, A. (1994). *Human cytogenetics database*. Oxford University Press, Oxford.

Schinzel, A. (2001). *Catalogue of unbalanced chromosome aberrations in man*, 2nd ed. Walter de Gruyter, Berlin.

10

Other Mechanisms
of Inheritance

It is conventional to consider genetic disorders under the headings of chromosomal, single-gene (autosomal dominant, autosomal recessive, X-linked recessive), multifactorial, and acquired. While most disorders encountered at a genetics clinic can be classified under one of these headings, there is increasing recognition that occasionally an alternative genetic mechanism should be considered that could often have significant implications for genetic counseling. In this chapter, some of these more unusual genetic mechanisms will be discussed and, where appropriate, due attention given to the relevant implications for risk calculation.

10.1 X-Linked Dominant Inheritance

A disorder that shows X-linked dominant inheritance is manifest both in the hemizygous male and in the heterozygous female. The disorder is transmitted on the X chromosome, so that an affected heterozygous female transmits the condition on average to half of her sons and to half of her daughters. In contrast, an affected male transmits the disorder to all of his daughters and to none of his sons. Consequently, male-to-male transmission does not occur. If affected males and females show normal fertility, then the incidence in females will be approximately twice the incidence in males, as females possess two X chromosomes. Generally, males are more severely affected than females because of the protection afforded to females by X-chromosome inactivation. Examples of disorders showing X-linked dominant inheritance are given in Table 10.1.

Table 10.1. Disorders Showing X-Linked Dominant Inheritance

Males More Severely Affected Than Females

Aarskog syndrome (305400)
Alport syndrome (301050)
Coffin-Lowry syndrome (303600)
Frontometaphyseal dysplasia (305620)
Ornithine transcarbamylase deficiency (311250)
Oto-palato-digital syndrome type 1 (311300)
Osteopathia striata with cranial sclerosis (300373)
Pyruvate decarboxylase deficiency (312170)
Subcortical laminar heterotopia/X-linked lissencephaly (300067)
Vitamin D–resistant rickets (307800)

Lethal in Affected Males

Affected females are able to reproduce
Chondrodysplasia punctata (302960)
Focal dermal hypoplasia (Goltz syndrome) (305600)
Incontinentia pigmenti (308300)
Melnick-Needles syndrome (309350)
Oral-facial-digital syndrome type 1 (311200)
Periventricular heterotopia (300049)
Affected females rarely reproduce
Aicardi syndrome (304050)
MLS (MIDAS) syndrome (309801)
Rett syndrome (312750)

Males Not Affected

Craniofrontonasal dysplasia (304110)
Epilepsy with mental retardation (EFMR) (300088)

Numbers in parentheses refer to entries in OMIM (Online Mendelian Inheritance in Man). McKusick-Nathans Institute for Genetic Medicine, Johns Hopkins University (Baltimore), and the National Center for Biotechnology Information, National Library of Medicine (Bethesda, MD), 2000. URL: http://www.ncbi.nlm.nih.gov/omim.

Key Point 1

In X-linked dominant inheritance an affected male transmits the disorder to all of his daughters and to none of his sons. An affected female transmits the disorder on average to half of her daughters and to half of her sons.

10.2 X-Linked Dominant Inheritance with Male Lethality

In some X-linked dominant disorders the male is so severely affected that survival is very unusual (Table 10.1). If a heterozygous female is able to reproduce, her surviving offspring will consist of affected females, unaffected females, and unaffected males in a ratio of 1:1:1. Overall this yields a male: female offspring ratio of

1:2. The very rare observation of isolated cases of live-born male infants with one of these disorders could be explained either by the presence of an additional X chromosome (i.e., Klinefelter syndrome—47,XXY) or by a mutation having occurred in only one half-strand of the DNA double helix. This latter phenomenon is referred to as a *half chromatid mutation* (Gartler and Francke, 1975).

Table 10.1 also includes several disorders in which the degree of severity is such that affected females rarely, if ever, reproduce. Unless a specific mutation can be identified in these disorders, it is not possible to conclude with confidence that they are, in fact, caused by X-chromosome mutations. Generally, it is believed that all observed cases of these disorders represent new mutations with a negligible risk to siblings and offspring of other family members. Rare examples of sibling recurrence can be explained by parental germline mosaicism.

Note that if the causal X-chromosome mutation occurs only in the male germline, as has been shown for several autosomal conditions such as achondroplasia and Apert syndrome, then all affected cases will be female. If the affected female is unable to reproduce, then there will never be any affected males. Thus, the absence of affected males with a specific X-linked condition could reflect the parental origin of new mutations rather than failure of affected males to survive (Thomas, 1996).

Key Point 2

A few disorders show X-linked dominant inheritance with male lethality. Affected females who reproduce show a male:female offspring ratio of 1:2.

10.3 X-Linked Dominant Inheritance with Male Sparing

Two disorders, craniofrontonasal dysplasia (CFND) and epilepsy with mental retardation limited to females (EFMR), show X-linked dominant inheritance with transmission through unaffected males. Male-to-male transmission does not occur, and almost all daughters born to unaffected transmitting males are affected. Both of these disorders have been mapped to the X chromosome (Feldman et al., 1997; Ryan et al., 1997), and the specific gene causing CFND has been identified (Twigg et al., 2004; Wieland et al., 2004). In CFND, transmitting males can show very mild clinical involvement, in contrast to affected females, who are usually much more severely affected. For transmitting males the risk to male offspring is negligible, whereas the risk to female offspring is very high—close to 100%. For affected females there is a probability of 50% that a daughter will be affected and that a son will be an unaffected hemizygote.

Despite the discovery of the gene Ephrin-B1, which causes CFND, the explanation for this curious pattern of male sparing is unclear. There is no homologue on the Y chromosome, and X-chromosome inactivation is normal. Wieland et al. (2004) propose that in heterozygous females there is an adverse interaction between Ephrin B1-positive and Ephrin B1-negative cells leading to disturbance of normal cell sorting and migration in early embryogenesis. Males are not affected, or show only very minor features, because their cell population is homogeneous for Ephrin B1 cells regardless of whether they are positive or negative. As these authors point out, this is reminiscent of the concept of metabolic interference.

10.4 Metabolic Interference

Metabolic interference was originally proposed by Johnson (1980) to explain how a disorder could occur exclusively in females or affect females much more severely than males. According to this theory, there are two alleles, A and B, at a locus on the X chromosome that code for slightly different forms or subunits of a structural protein. Homozygotes for the normal allele (AA) and the mutant allele (BB) have a normal phenotype. However, in the heterozygous state (AB), the different protein products interact to cause an abnormal phenotype so that only the heterozygote is affected (Fig. 10.1).

According to this hypothesis, abnormalities would only be observed in females since the male is hemizygous. The condition would be passed on by males, who might show minor features. X-chromosome inactivation would not prevent manifestation in a heterozygous female if the gene is expressed in tissues with multinucleate cells. Alternatively, the gene could encode a protein that is secreted into the extracellular space to form a dimer with its allelic product or, as in CFND, is an important factor in determining how different populations of cells recognize and interact with each other. As an alternative to metabolic interference, Wieland et al. (2004) propose that this phenomenon be referred to as *cellular* interference. Mechanistically this is similar to the principle underlying the concept of dominant negative mutations whereby the product of a mutant allele interferes with the function or product of the normal wild-type allele, possibly by leading to the formation of an abnormal multimeric protein.

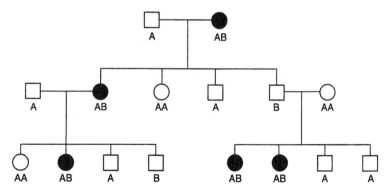

Figure 10.1. The mechanism underlying the theory of metabolic interference. A and B represent alleles at a locus on the X chromosome. A is the common wild-type allele; B is a rare mutant allele. Interaction between the A and B gene products results in an abnormal phenotype.

The concept of metabolic interference could also apply to autosomal loci. In this situation, individuals who are homozygous for a mutant dominant allele would be unaffected, in contrast to the usual situation in which they are more severely affected than heterozygotes (p. 35). Primary open-angle glaucoma is a very rare example of a disorder in which this phenomenon has been observed (Morissette et al., 1998).

Key Point 3

Two rare disorders, CFND and EFMR, show X-linked inheritance with only females affected. One possible explanation is that heterozygotes are affected because of metabolic or cellular interference, whereas homozygotes and hemizygotes are unaffected.

10.5 Digenic Inheritance

Digenic inheritance can be defined formally as the pattern of inheritance that results from the interaction of genes at two loci. There is clear evidence from studies in mice that some neural tube defects are caused by digenic inheritance through an interaction between mutations in *Pax1* and the platelet-derived growth factor alpha gene (*Pdgfra*). Similarly, mice heterozygous for both the curly tail (*ct*) and SPLOTCH (*Pax3*) mutations show a higher incidence of neural tube defects than is seen in either heterozygote alone (Estibeiro et al., 1993). In humans, digenic inheritance was first demonstrated in several kindreds with retinitis pigmentosa (Kajiwara et al., 1994). The fact that this inheritance pattern has now been recognized in several other disorders (Table 10.2) suggests that it may be a relatively common occurrence.

Digenic inheritance can be suspected when unaffected, unrelated parents have multiple affected offspring, who then transmit the disorder to approximately 25% of their offspring. The hypothesis is that the parents in the first generation are heterozygous for a recessive mutation at two different loci. These encode products that either form a molecular or protein complex or are involved in the same

Table 10.2. Disorders in Which Digenic Inheritance Has Been Demonstrated

Disorder	Reference
Hemochromatosis	Merryweather-Clarke et al. (2003)
Insulin resistance	Savage et al. (2002)
Primary congenital glaucoma	Kaur et al. (2005)
Retinitis pigmentosa	Kajiwara et al. (1994)
Sensorineural hearing loss	Lerer et al. (2001)
Usher syndrome	Xheng et al. (2005)

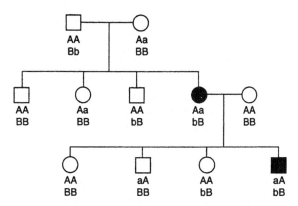

Figure 10.2. The mechanism underlying digenic inheritance. Aa and Bb represent wild-type and mutant alleles at two loci. Double heterozygosity for the recessive alleles a and b results in an abnormal phenotype.

developmental or metabolic pathway. Only offspring who inherit both of the recessive nonallelic mutations are affected, so that the segregation ratio in the first generation is 25%. For these affected members of the first generation, who are essentially double heterozygotes, there will be 1 chance in 4 that they will transmit both of their mutant alleles to their own offspring, so that once again the segregation ratio is 25%. This assumes that the relevant loci are not linked. This mechanism is illustrated in Figure 10.2. Note that this pattern of inheritance is similar to that which would be expected for an autosomal dominant disorder showing reduced penetrance of 50%.

The Bardet-Biedl syndrome demonstrates a different form of digenic inheritance in that in a few families it is caused by the combined effects of homozygous mutations at one locus and a heterozygous mutation at another locus (Katsanis et al., 2001). This requirement for the presence of three mutations has been referred to as *triallelic* inheritance. In this situation the recurrence risk for parents with one affected child is 1 in 8 (i.e. $1/4 \times 1/2$). The probability that an affected individual would transmit the disorder to his or her offspring is very low.

Key Point 4

Digenic inheritance has been demonstrated in a small number of disorders caused by double heterozygosity for recessive mutations at different loci. In these families the risk to offspring in each generation is 1 in 4. In triallelic inheritance the recurrence risk for parents of an affected child is 1 in 8.

10.6 Uniparental Disomy and Genomic Imprinting

It is now well established that a small proportion of the human genome shows differential expression, depending on the parent of origin. This memory or *imprint* of parental origin is thought to be achieved by differential DNA methylation.

The parental imprint persists through DNA replication and cell division in the embryo and throughout life, but is removed during gametogenesis and then reestablished according to whether transmission occurs in the sperm or the egg. This phenomenon of imprinting can have important implications for the transmission and expression of genetic disease in humans and should be considered as a possible explanation for an inheritance pattern that does not show strict adherence to Mendelian laws. Several mechanisms have been identified that can reveal an imprinting effect. These are discussed in the context of the Angelman and Prader-Willi syndromes.

Microdeletion

If a microdeletion occurs de novo in a critical region of the paternally inherited chromosome 15, this results in the child developing the Prader-Willi syndrome. Conversely, if the deletion occurs de novo in a similar region of the maternally inherited chromosome 15, then the child develops Angelman syndrome. The explanation for these curious observations is that the chromosome region 15q11-q13 contains a cluster of genes that show parent-specific imprinting determined by a bipartite imprinting center. Absence of the paternally derived imprinted genes or failure of normal expression of the paternal imprint center causes the Prader-Willi syndrome; absence of the maternally imprinted genes or abnormal expression of the maternal imprint center causes Angelman syndrome.

Uniparental Disomy

This refers to the presence in an individual of two homologous chromosomes derived from a single parent. The presence of two copies of one homologue is referred to as *uniparental isodisomy*. In theory, this can arise as a result of nondisjunction in meiosis II. If the original error in nondisjunction has occurred in meiosis I, then the gamete will acquire both copies of that parent's homologues, and if this gamete is then fertilized, this will lead to *uniparental heterodisomy*. In practice, there is usually a mixture of isodisomy and heterodisomy because of recombination. A disomic gamete would be expected to result in a trisomic conceptus, and for most of the human autosomes the outcome will be early spontaneous pregnancy loss. However, early loss of a chromosome from the trisomic conceptus (*trisomy rescue*) would result in restoration of the normal disomic state, and the pregnancy would survive. In this event, there is 1 chance in 3 that the chromsome transmitted in the monosomic gamete will have been lost, resulting in the surviving embryo having uniparental disomy (UPD) (Fig. 10.3). Alternative explanations for UPD include *monosomy rescue*, in which a monosomic conceptus survives due to postzygotic duplication of the single copy of the relevant chromosome, and *gamete complementation*, in which fertilization occurs between nullisomic and disomic gametes.

Often UPD will have no clinical significance. However, if part of the relevant chromosome is imprinted, then the surviving child will not have received normally imprinted genes from both parents. Uniparental disomy has been shown to account for approximately 25% of children with Prader-Willi syndrome and 2%–3% of children with Angelman syndrome. Other clinically important outcomes associated with UPD are summarized in Table 10.3.

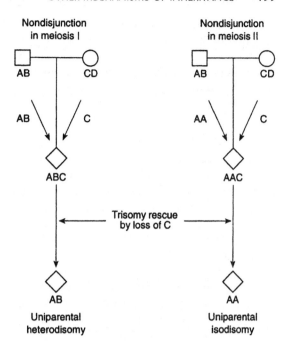

Figure 10.3. The origin of uniparental heterodisomy and uniparental isodisomy. A, B, C, and D represent the parental homologous chromosomes.

Uniparental disomy can also cause medical problems by doubling up a mutant recessive allele from one of the parents, resulting in a child being affected with an autosomal recessive disorder despite having only one carrier parent. Coinheritance of the X and Y chromosomes from a father to son provides a unique mechanism for male-to-male transmission of an X-linked disorder and accounts for rare reports of male-to-male transmission of X-linked disorders such as hemophilia.

Table 10.3. Clinical Outcome of UPD for an Imprinted Chromosome

Chromosome	Parental Origin	Outcome
6	Paternal	Transient neonatal diabetes mellitus and low birth weight
7	Maternal	Silver-Russell syndrome
11	Paternal	Beckwith-Wiedemann syndrome
14	Paternal	Short stature with small chest, facial dysmorphism, and mental retardation
	Maternal	Pre- and postnatal growth retardation, obesity, and precocious puberty
15	Paternal	Angelman syndrome
	Maternal	Prader-Willi syndrome
16	Maternal	Severe IUGR, variable malformations, and short stature

IUGR, intrauterine growth retardation; UPD, uniparental disomy. For further details see Engel and Antonarakis (2002) and Kotzot and Utermann (2005).

The recurrence risk for UPD will usually be extremely small, with the possible exception of Robertsonian translocations (p. 174). The finding of true placental mosaicism for trisomy of an imprinted chromosome at prenatal diagnosis presents a very difficult counseling problem, as it conveys a risk of 1 in 3 for UPD in a surviving disomic infant. In these situations, molecular analysis is indicated to determine the parental origin of the chromosomes in the fetus.

Imprinting Mutation

In a small number of families, a point mutation or small deletion has been identified that prevents normal expression of one part of the bipartite imprinting center located at 15q11-q13. Awareness of this possibility is important when counseling families in which a child with the Prader-Willi or Angelman syndrome does not have a microdeletion or UPD. For example, if the father of a child with unexplained Prader-Willi syndrome has inherited from his mother a point mutation that prevents normal expression of the paternal imprinting center, then there will be 1 chance in 2 that he will transmit this mutant allele to each of his children, who will therefore be affected (Fig. 10.4). The father himself is not affected because he has inherited a perfectly normal paternal imprint center from his father. Similarly, if a woman inherits from her father a mutation in the maternal imprint center, or in the exclusively maternally expressed gene *UBE3A*, then there is 1 chance in 2 that she will transmit this to each of her children, who will be affected with Angelman syndrome. The woman is not affected because she has inherited a normal maternal imprint center from her mother. In these rare situations the recurrence risk for offspring will be 1 in 2.

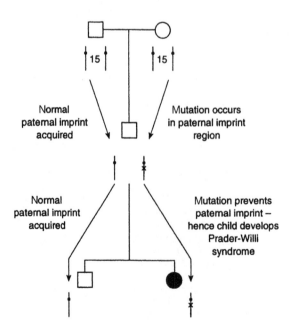

Figure 10.4. The mechanism underlying inheritance of an imprinting mutation resulting in the Prader-Willi syndrome.

Key Point 5

A small proportion of the human genome shows differential parental imprinting. This can become manifest if a de novo microdeletion involves an imprinted region or if there is UPD for an imprinted chromosome. In these situations the recurrence risk will usually be very low. If an imprinting disorder such as Angelman or Prader-Willi syndrome has been caused by a mutation that prevents normal expression of an imprinting center or of an imprinted gene, then the recurrence risk will be 1 in 2 if the mutation is present in the relevant parent.

10.7 Somatic Crossing-Over

Crossing-over (recombination) in meiosis and its implications for risk calculation were considered at length in Chapter 5. Crossing-over can also occur between homologous chromosomes during mitosis in somatic cells (Therman and Kuhn, 1981) and provides one possible explanation for a recessive mutant allele becoming homozygous in a single cell, with pathological consequences in all daughter cells. Thus, if an individual is heterozygous at a particular locus with alleles A and a, then somatic crossing-over between two of the nonsister chromatids could lead to one daughter cell with genotype AA and the other daughter cell with genotype aa (Fig. 10.5).

Evidence for the occurrence of somatic crossing-over in plants and *Drosophila* is well established, with the classical example being the *twin-spot* phenomenon, which has been used as a test marker for recombinogenic activity of potentially toxic substances. In a very simple system there are two alleles, A and B, coding for dark and light skin, respectively. An AB genotype results in an intermediate skin color. If somatic recombination occurs in an AB cell, resulting in daughter cells with AA and BB genotypes, this will be distinguishable as an area of increased skin pigmentation closely adjacent to an area of decreased skin pigmentation.

Key Point 6

Somatic crossing-over in a constitutional heterozygote can result in a recessive allele becoming homozygous in somatic cells. This, in turn, can lead to tumor formation, as in hereditary retinoblastoma, or to partial UPD, as in the Beckwith-Wiedemann syndrome.

Somatic crossing-over can play an important role in humans in the genesis of tumors such as retinoblastoma (Cavenee et al., 1983) by facilitating homozygosity for a recessive allele. This is one possible explanation for how a disease that shows dominant inheritance is actually caused by a recessive mechanism at a cellular level. Somatic recombination can also result in partial UPD, and if the relevant

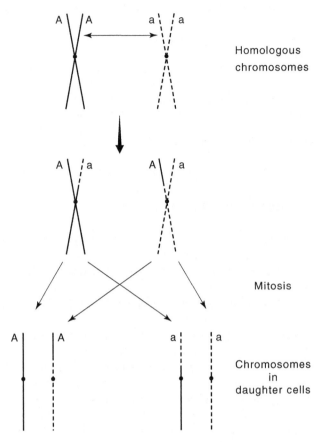

Figure 10.5. Diagrammatic representation of somatic crossing-over between homologous chromosomes resulting in daughter cells that are homozygous and show partial UPD. The horizontal arrow shows the site of recombination.

chromosome region is imprinted, this can cause one of the recognized imprinting syndromes. Postzygotic mitotic crossing-over involving chromosome 11p accounts for approximately 10%–20% of cases of the Beckwith-Wiedemann syndrome.

10.8 Meiotic Drive

Meiotic drive is the term used to describe segregation distortion caused by preferential transmission of one of a pair of alleles during meiosis. Essentially this means that a specific allele is transmitted significantly more or less often than would be expected according to traditional Mendelian inheritance, i.e., in more or less than 50% of gametes. This phenomenon of a "selfish" allele or chromosome has been observed in *Drosophila* and mice, but its existence in humans is much less certain.

Table 10.4. Human Disorders Reported to Show Meiotic Drive

Disorder	Transmitting Sex	Confirmed
Cone-rod retinal dystrophy (Evans et al., 1994)	Female	No data
Dentatorubral-pallidoluysian atrophy (Ikeuchi et al., 1996)	Male	No (Takiyama et al., 1999)
Ectrodactyly (Jarvik et al., 1994)	Male	No data
Machado-Joseph disease (Ikeuchi et al., 1996)	Male	No (Grewal et al., 1999)
Myotonic dystrophy (Carey et al., 1994; Shaw et al., 1995)	Male and female	No (Leeflang et al., 1996; Zunc et al., 2004)
Retinoblastoma (Munier et al., 1992)	Male	No (Girardet et al., 2000)

The classic example of meiotic drive is that of the t haplotype in mice. During spermatogenesis in heterozygous males, spermatids with the t haplotype suppress development of t haplotype-negative spermatids, resulting in almost all of the mature sperm being t haplotype-positive. The t haplotype is generated by genes at four or more closely linked loci, which segregate together because of a series of inversions that suppress crossing-over. An equally complex mechanism accounts for the segregation-distortion (SD) system seen in *Drosophila* (Charlesworth, 1988).

This complexity probably explains why meiotic drive appears to be extremely rare in humans. There have been suggestions that several conditions, particularly those caused by triplet repeat expansions (Hurst et al., 1995), demonstrate this phenomenon, but independent confirmation has not been forthcoming for any of these (Table 10.4). However, the demonstration of meiotic drive in other species, such as *Drosophila* and mice, suggests that due consideration should be given to this possibility if a disorder consistently shows a segregation ratio that differs significantly from that to be expected according to traditional Mendelian inheritance.

10.9 Mitochondrial Inheritance

While the vast majority of DNA is contained within the nucleus, a very small quantity is also found in each mitochondrion. This consists of approximately 16.5 kilobases encoding 13 polypeptides, all of which are components of the mitochondrial respiratory chain and the oxidative phosphorylation system, as well as two ribosomal RNAs and 22 transfer RNAs. Mitochondrial disorders can result from (1) maternally inherited mutations, deletions, or duplications in mitochondrial DNA, (2) nuclear mutations that alter the integrity of the mitochondrial genome, (3) nuclear mutations that impair oxidative phosphorylation, or (4) acquired mitochondrial DNA rearrangements. The accumulation of somatically acquired mitochondrial DNA rearrangements is thought to be a major contributory factor to the process of aging.

These diverse causes of mitochondrial disease mean that in practice it is often very difficult to determine risks for other family members. The importance of identifying a germline mitochondrial DNA point mutation rests in the almost exclusive inheritance of mitochondria from the female. Human ova contain approximately 100,000 mitochondria, whereas sperm contains fewer than 100, almost all of which are selectively eliminated following conception. Thus mitochondrial inheritance is unique in that transmission occurs exclusively though the female. This means that the offspring of an affected male can be confidently reassured. It is usually much more difficult to give accurate information to the offspring or collateral relatives of an affected female. Risks can be influenced by the nature of the underlying mutation, by whether it is present in some or all mitochondria (heteroplasmy or homoplasmy), and by the proportion of mitochondria in which the mutation is present in different tissues. In theory, it could be possible to determine risks to offspring by analyzing mitochondrial DNA in oocytes obtained at IVF, but in practice this is rarely feasible.

Key Point 7

Mitochondria are inherited exclusively through the female line. Therefore, the probability that an affected male will transmit a mitochondrial mutation to his offspring is extremely low. Risks for the offspring of affected or carrier females are much more difficult to determine but can sometimes be obtained from the results of empiric family studies. Major rearrangements in mitochondrial DNA generally convey much lower risks than point mutations.

For some mitochondrial disorders it is possible to use empiric recurrence risks obtained from relatively large family studies. For example, Harding et al. (1995) derived recurrence risks of 30%, 8%, 46%, 10%, 31%, and 6%, respectively, for the brothers, sisters, nephews, nieces, and male and female matrilineal first cousins of index cases with Leber's hereditary optic neuropathy (LHON). However, even for this disorder, which has been studied intensely, it can be difficult to give accurate risk information, as the penetrance of the different pathogenic mutations differs and it is still not understood why the male is much more susceptible than the female. Poulton et al. (2003) have provided useful guidelines for risk estimation and prenatal diagnosis for mitochondrial disorders in general. As a rough rule of thumb, major rearrangements—as seen, for example, in the Kearns-Sayre syndrome—are usually acquired sporadically and convey low recurrence risks to other family members. In contrast, point mutations in mitochondrial DNA, which account for disorders such as LHON and the mitochondrial encephalomyopathy, lactic acidosis, and stroke-like symptoms (MELAS), myoclonus epilepsy with ragged red fibers (MERRF), and neurodegeneration, ataxia and retinitis pigmentosa (NARP) syndromes, convey high risks for offspring and matrilineal relatives. These risks tend to correlate with the proportion of mutant DNA present in maternal blood but with wide confidence intervals (Chinnery et al., 1998; White et al., 1999).

Further Reading

Engel, E. and Antonarakis, S.E. (2002). *Genomic imprinting and uniparental disomy in medicine.* Wiley-Liss, New York.

Holt, I.J. (Ed). (2003). *Genetics of mitochondrial disease.* Oxford University Press, Oxford.

Kotzot, D. and Utermann, U. (2005). Uniparental disomy (UPD) other than 15: phenotypes and bibliography updated. *American Journal of Medical Genetics,* **136A,** 287–305.

Ming, J.E. and Muenke, M. (2002). Multiple hits during early embryonic development: digenic diseases and holoprosencephaly. *American Journal of Human Genetics,* **71,** 1017–1032.

Wettke-Schäfer, R. and Kantner, G. (1983). X-linked dominant inherited diseases with lethality in hemizygous males. *Human Genetics,* **64,** 1–23.

References

Anton, E., Blanco, J., Egozcue, J., and Vidal, F. (2005). Sperm studies in heterozygote inversion carriers: a review. *Cytogenetic and Genome Research*, **111**, 297–304.

Antoniou, A., Pharoah, P.D.P., Narod, S., et al. (2003). Average risks of breast and ovarian cancer associated with *BRCA1* or *BRCA2* mutations detected in case series unselected for family history: a combined analysis of 22 studies. *American Journal of Human Genetics*, **72**, 1117–1130.

Aylsworth, A.S. and Kirkman, H.N. (1979). Genetic counselling for autosomal dominant disorders with incomplete penetrance. In *Risk, communication, and decision making in genetic counseling* (ed. C.J. Epstein, C.J.R. Curry, S. Packman, S. Sherman, and B.D. Hall), Birth Defects: Original Article Series, Vol. XV (5C), pp. 25–38. Alan R. Liss, Inc., New York, for the National Foundation–March of Dimes.

Ayukawa, H., Tsukahara, M., Fukuda, M., and Kondoh, O. (1994). Recombinant chromosome 18 resulting from a maternal pericentric inversion. *American Journal of Medical Genetics*, **50**, 323–325.

Bakker, K., Veenema, H., Den Dunnen, J.T., et al. (1989). Germinal mosaicism increases the recurrence risk for "new" Duchenne muscular dystrophy mutations. *Journal of Medical Genetics*, **26**, 553–559.

Barisic, I., Zergollern, L., Muzinic, D., and Hitrec, V. (1996). Risk estimates for balanced reciprocal translocation carriers—prenatal diagnosis experience. *Clinical Genetics*, **49**, 145–151.

Batista, D.A.S., Pai, G.S., and Stetton, G. (1994). Molecular analysis of a complex chromosomal rearrangement and a review of familial cases. *American Journal of Medical Genetics*, **53**, 255–263.

Bayes, T. (1958). An essay towards solving a problem in the doctrine of chances. *Biometrika*, **45**, 296–315.

Beaudet, A.L., Feldman, G.L., Fernbach, S.D., Buffone, G.J., and O'Brien, W.E. (1989). Linkage disequilibrium, cystic fibrosis, and genetic counseling. *American Journal of Human Genetics*, **44**, 319–326.

Becker, J., Schwaab, R., Möller-Taube, A. et al. (1996). Characterization of the Factor VIII defect in 147 patients with sporadic hemophilia A: family studies indicate a mutation type-dependent sex ratio of mutation frequencies. *American Journal of Human Genetics*, **58,** 657–670.

Benet, J., Oliver-Bonet, M., Cifuentes, P., Templado, C., and Navarro, J. (2005). Segregation of chromosomes in sperm of reciprocal translocation carriers: a review. *Cytogenetic and Genome Research*, **111,** 281–290.

Berry, D.A., Iversen, E.S., Gudbjartsson, D.F., et al. (2002). BRCAPRO validation, sensitivity of genetic testing of *BRCA1/BRCA2*, and prevalence of other breast cancer susceptibility genes. *Journal of Clinical Oncology*, **20,** 2701–2712.

Bittles, A.H. and Neel, J.V. (1994). The costs of human inbreeding and their implications at the DNA level. *Nature Genetics*, **8,** 117–121.

Blackwood, M.A., Yang, H., Margolin, A., et al. (2001). Predicted probability of breast cancer susceptibility gene mutations. *Breast Cancer Research and Treatment*, **69,** 223–229.

Bonaiti, C. (1978). Genetic counselling of consanguineous families. *Journal of Medical Genetics*, **15,** 109–112.

Bonaiti-Pellié, C. and Smith, C. (1974). Risk tables for genetic counselling in some common congenital malformations. *Journal of Medical Genetics*, **11,** 374–377.

Bosco, A., Norton, M.E., and Lieberman, E. (1999). Predicting the risk of cystic fibrosis with echogenic fetal bowel and one cystic fibrosis mutation. *Obstetrics and Gynecology*, **94,** 1020–1023.

Boué, A. and Gallano, P. (1984). A collaborative study of the segregation of inherited chromosome structural rearrangements in 1356 prenatal diagnoses. *Prenatal Diagnosis*, **4,** 45–67.

Bremner R., Du, D.C., Connolly-Wilson, M.J., et al., (1997). Deletion of *RB* exons 24 and 25 causes low-penetrance retinoblastoma. *American Journal of Human Genetics*, **61,** 556–570.

Burn, J., Chapman, P., Wood, C., et al. (1991). The UK Northern Region genetic register for FAP: use of age of onset, CHRPE and DNA markers in risk calculations. *Journal of Medical Genetics*, **28,** 289–296.

Byers, P.H., Tsipouras, P., Bonadio, J.F., Starman, B.J., and Schwartz, R.C. (1988). Perinatal lethal osteogenesis imperfecta (OI type II): a biochemically heterogeneous disorder usually due to new mutations in the genes for type I collagen. *American Journal of Human Genetics*, **42,** 237–248.

Cans, C., Cohen, O., Lavergne, C., et al. (1993). Logistic regression model to estimate the risk of unbalanced offspring in reciprocal translocations. *Human Genetics* **92,** 598–604.

Carey, N., Johnson, K., Nokelainen, P., et al. (1994). Meiotic drive at the myotonic dystrophy locus? *Nature Genetics*, **6,** 117–118.

Carter, C.O. (1961). The inheritance of congenital pyloric stenosis. *British Medical Bulletin*, **17,** 251–254.

Carter, C.O., Evans, K., Coffey, R., Fraser-Roberts, J.A., Buck, A., and Fraser-Roberts, M. (1982). A three generation family study of cleft lip with or without cleft palate. *Journal of Medical Genetics*, **19,** 246–261.

Cavenee, W.K., Dryja, T.P., Phillips, R.A., et al. (1983). Expression of recessive alleles by chromosomal mechanisms in retinoblastoma. *Nature*, **305,** 779–784.

Charlesworth, B. (1988). Driving genes and chromosomes. *Nature*, **332,** 394–395.

Chinnery, P.F., Howell, N., Lightowlers, R.N., and Turnbull, D.M. (1998). MELAS and MERRF. The relationship between maternal mutation load and the frequency of clinically affected offspring. *Brain*, **121,** 1889–1894.

Cifuentes, P., Navarro, J., Míguez L., Egozcue, J., and Benet, J. (1998). Sperm segregation analysis of a complex chromosome rearrangement, 2;22;11, by whole chromosome painting. *Cytogenetics and Cell Genetics*, **82,** 204–209.

Claus, E.B., Risch, N.J., and Thompson, W.D. (1990). Age at onset as an indicator of familial risk of breast cancer. *American Journal of Epidemiology*, **131**, 961–972.

Claus, E.B., Risch, N., and Thompson, W.D. (1993). The calculation of breast cancer risk for women with a first degree family history of ovarian cancer. *Breast Cancer Research and Treatment*, **28**, 115–120.

Claus, E.B., Risch, N., and Thompson, W.D. (1994). Autosomal dominant inheritance of early-onset breast cancer: implications for risk prediction. *Cancer*, **73**, 643–651.

Cohen, O., Cans, C., Mermet, M., Demongeot, J., and Jalbert, P. (1994). Viability thresholds for partial trisomies and monosomies. A study of 1,159 viable unbalanced reciprocal translocations. *Human Genetics*, **93**, 188–194.

Cohn, D.H., Starman, B.J., Blumberg, B., and Byers, P.H. (1990). Recurrence of lethal osteogenesis imperfecta due to parental mosaicism for a dominant mutation in a human type I collagen gene (COLIAI). *American Journal of Human Genetics*, **46**, 591–601.

Couch, F.J., DeShano, M.L., Blackwood, M.A., et al. (1997). *BRCA1* mutations in women attending clinics that evaluate the risk of breast cancer. *New England Journal of Medicine*, **336**, 1409–1415.

Crow, J.F. (2000). The origins, patterns and implications of human spontaneous mutation. *Nature Reviews*, **1**, 40–47.

Curnow, R.N. (1972). The multifactorial model for the inheritance of liability to disease and its implications for relatives at risk. *Biometrics*, **28**, 931–946.

Curnow, R.N. (1994). Carrier risk calculations for recessive diseases when not all the mutant alleles are detectable. *American Journal of Medical Genetics*, **52**, 108–114.

Daniel, A. (1979). Structural differences in reciprocal translocations. Potential for a model of risk in rcp. *Human Genetics*, **51**, 171–182.

Daniel, A. (1981). Structural differences in pericentric inversions. Application to a model of risk of recombinants. *Human Genetics*, **56**, 321–328.

Daniel, A. (1985). The size of prometaphase chromosome segments. *Clinical Genetics*, **28**, 216–224.

Daniel, A., Hook, E.B., and Wulf, G. (1988). Collaborative USA data on prenatal diagnosis for parental carriers of chromosome rearrangements: risks of unbalanced progeny. In *The cytogenetics of mammalian autosomal rearrangements* (ed. A. Daniel), pp. 73–162. Alan R. Liss, New York.

Dennis, N.R. and Carter, C.O. (1978). Use of overlapping normal distributions in genetic counselling. *Journal of Medical Genetics*, **15**, 106–108.

Doheny, K.F., Rasmussen, S.A., Rutberg, J., et al. (1997). Segregation of a familial balanced (12;10) insertion resulting in dup (10)(q21.2q22.1) and del (10)(q21.2q22.1) in first cousins. *American Journal of Medical Genetics*, **69**, 188–193.

Easton, D.F., Ponder, M.A., Huson, S.M., and Ponder, B.A.J. (1993). An analysis of variation in expression of NFI: evidence for modifying genes. *American Journal of Medical Genetics*, **53**, 305–313.

Eccles, D.M., Evans, D.G.R., and Mackay, J. (2000). Guidelines for a genetic risk based approach to advising women with a family history of breast cancer. *Journal of Medical Genetics*, **37**, 204–209.

Edwards, J.H. (1969). Familial predisposition in man. *British Medical Bulletin*, **25**, 58–64.

Edwards, J.H. (1976). Risks of malformed relatives. *Lancet*, **1**, 1348.

Edwards, J.H. (1989). Familiarity, recessivity and germline mosaicism. *Annals of Human Genetics*, **53**, 33–47.

Emery, A.E.H. (1986). Risk estimation in autosomal dominant disorders with reduced penetrance. *Journal of Medical Genetics*, **23**, 316–318.

Emery, A.E.H. (1997). Duchenne and other X-linked muscular dystrophies. In *Principles and practice of medical genetics* 3rd. ed. (ed. D.L. Rimoin, J.M. Connor, and R.E. Pyeritz), pp. 2337–2354. Churchill Livingstone, New York.

Emery, A.E.H. and Lawrence, J.S. (1967). Genetics of ankylosing spondylitis. *Journal of Medical Genetics*, **4**, 239–244.

Estibeiro, J.P., Brook, F.A., and Copp, A.J. (1993). Interaction between splotch (Sp) and curly tail (ct) mouse mutants in the embryonic development of neural tube defects. *Development*, **119**, 113–121.

Evans, D.G.R., Eccles, D.M., Rahman, N., et al. (2004). A new scoring system for the chances of identifying a *BRCA1/2* mutation outperforms existing models including BRCAPRO. *Journal of Medical Genetics*, **41**, 474–480.

Evans, K., Fryer, A., Inglehearn, C., et al. (1994). Genetic linkage of cone-rod retinal dystrophy to chromosome 19q and evidence for segregation distortion. *Nature Genetics*, **6**, 210–213.

Falace, P., Ruderman, R.J., Ward, F.E., and Swift, M. (1978). Histocompatibility typing and the counseling of families with ankylosing spondylitis. *Clinical Genetics*, **13**, 380–383.

Falconer, D.S. (1965). The inheritance of liability to certain diseases, estimated from the incidence among relatives. *Annals of Human Genetics*, **29**, 51–76.

Feldman, G.J., Ward, D.E., Lajeunie-Renier, E., et al. (1997). A novel phenotypic pattern in X-linked inheritance: craniofrontonasal syndrome maps to Xp22. *Human Molecular Genetics*, **6**, 1937–1941.

Ferrie, R.M., Schwartz, M.J., Robertson, N.H., et al. (1992). Development, multiplexing, and application of ARMS tests for common mutations in the *CFTR* gene. *American Journal of Human Genetics*, **51**, 251–262.

Firth, H.V. and Hurst, J.A. (2005). *Oxford desk reference, clinical genetics.* Oxford University Press, Oxford.

Flodman, P. and Hodge, S.E. (2002). Determining complex genetic risks by computer. *Journal of Genetic Counseling.* **11**, 213–230.

Flodman, P. and Hodge, S.E. (2003). Sex-specific mutation rates for X-linked disorders: estimation and application. *Human Heredity*, **55**, 51–55.

Ford, D., Easton, D.F., Stratton, M., et al. (1998). Genetic heterogeneity and penetrance analysis of the *BRCA1* and *BRCA2* genes in breast cancer families. *American Journal of Human Genetics*, **62**, 676–689.

Francke, U., Felsenstein, J., Gartler, S.M., et al. (1976). The occurrence of new mutants in the X-linked recessive Lesch-Nyhan disease. *American Journal of Human Genetics*, **28**, 123–137.

Frank, T.S., Deffenbaugh, A.M., Sanchez, J., et al. (2002). Clinical characteristics of individuals with germline mutations in *BRCA1* and *BRCA2:* analysis of 10,000 individuals. *Journal of Clinical Oncology*, **20**, 1480–1490.

Frank, T.S., Manley, S.A., Olopade, O.I., et al. (1998). Correlation of mutations with family history and ovarian cancer risk. *Journal of Clinical Oncology*, **16**, 2417–2425.

Fraser, F.C. (1980). Evolution of a palatable multifactorial threshold model. *American Journal of Human Genetics*, **32**, 796–813.

Friedman, J.M. (1985). Genetic counseling for autosomal dominant diseases with a negative family history. *Clinical Genetics*, **27**, 68–71.

Friedman, J.M. and Fish, R.D. (1980). The use of probability trees in genetic counselling. *Clinical Genetics*, **18**, 408–412.

Gardner, R.J.M. and Sutherland, G.R. *Chromosome abnormalities and genetic counseling*, 3rd ed. Oxford University Press, New York.

Gartler, S.M. and Francke, U. (1975). Half chromatid mutations: transmission in humans? *American Journal of Human Genetics*, **27**, 218–223.

Gianaroli, L., Magli, M.C., Ferraretti, A.P., et al. (2002). Possible interchromosomal effect in embryos generated by gametes from translocation carriers. *Human Reproduction*, **17**, 3201–3207.

Girardet, A., McPeek, M.S., Leeflang, E.P., et al. (2000). Meiotic segregation of RB1 alleles in retinoblastoma pedigrees by single-sperm typing. *American Journal of Human Genetics*, **66**, 167–175.

Gorski, J.L., Kistenmacher, M.L., Punnett, H.H., Zackai, E.H., and Emanuel, B.S. (1988). Reproductive risks for carriers of complex chromosome rearrangements: analysis of 25 families. *American Journal of Medical Genetics*, **29**, 247–261.

Gran, J.T. and Husby, G. (1995). HLA-B27 and spondyloarthropathy: value for early diagnosis. *Journal of Medical Genetics*, **32**, 497–501.

Green, P.M., Saad, S., Lewis, C.M., and Giannelli F. (1999). Mutation rates in humans. I. Overall and sex-specific rates obtained from a population study of hemophilia B. *American Journal of Human Genetics* **65**, 1572–1579.

Grewal, R.P., Cancel, G., Leeflang, E.P., et al. (1999). French Machado-Joseph disease patients do not exhibit gametic segregation distortion: a sperm typing analysis. *Human Molecular Genetics*, **8**, 1779–1784.

Grimm, T. (1984). Genetic counseling in Becker type X-linked muscular dystrophy. 1. Theoretical considerations. *American Journal of Medical Genetics*, **18**, 713–718.

Grimm, T., Meng, G., Liechti-Gallati, S., Bettecken, T., Müller C.R., and Müller B. (1994). On the origin of deletions and point mutations in Duchenne muscular dystrophy: most deletions arise in oogenesis and most point mutations result from events in spermatogenesis. *Journal of Medical Genetics*, **31**, 183–186.

Groupe de Cytogénéticiens Français, (1986a). Pericentric inversions in man. A French collaborative study. *Annales de Génétique*, **29**, 162–168.

Groupe de Cytogénéticiens Français, (1986b). Paracentric inversions in man. A French collaborative study. *Annales de Génétique*, **29**, 169–176.

Haldane, J.B.S. (1947). The mutation rate of the gene for haemophilia, and its segregation ratio in males and females. *Annals of Eugenics*, **13**, 262–271.

Haldane, J.B.S. (1949). The rate of mutation of human genes. *Hereditas (Suppl)*, **35**, 267–273.

Harding, A.E., Sweeney, M.G., Govan, G.G., and Riordan-Eva, P. (1995). Pedigree analysis in Leber hereditary optic neuropathy families with a pathogenic mtDNA mutation. *American Journal of Human Genetics*, **57**, 77–86.

Harper, P.S. and Newcombe, R.G. (1992). Age at onset and life table risks in genetic counselling for Huntington's disease. *Journal of Medical Genetics*, **29**, 239–242.

Harris, D.J., Hankins, L., and Begleiter, M.L. (1979). Reproductive risk of t(13q14q) carriers: case report and review. *American Journal of Medical Genetics*, **3**, 175–181.

Hartl, D.L. (1971). Recurrence risks for germinal mosaics. *American Journal of Human Genetics*, **23**, 124–134.

Herman, G.E., Kopacz, K., Zhao, W., Mills, P.L., Metzenberg, A., and Das, S. (2002). Characterization of mutations in fifty North American patients with X-linked myotubular myopathy. *Human Mutation* **19**, 114–121.

Hodge, S.E. and Flodman, P.L. (2004). Risk calculations: Still essential in the molecular age. *American Journal of Medical Genetics*, **129A**, 215–217.

Hodge, S.E. and Flodman, P.L. (2005). Re: "Risk calculations: Still essential in the molecular age," AJMG 129A:215–217. *American Journal of Medical Genetics*, **134A**, 112.

Hodge, S.E., Lebo, R.V., Yesley, A.R., et al. (1999). Calculating posterior cystic fibrosis risk with echogenic bowel and one characterized cystic fibrosis mutation: avoiding pitfalls in the risk calculations. *American Journal of Medical Genetics*, **82**, 329–335.

Hopwood, P., Howell, A., Lalloo, F., and Evans, G. (2003). Do women understand the odds? Risk perceptions and recall of risk information in women with a family history of breast cancer. *Community Genetics*, **6**, 214–223.

Huang, W., Qiu, C., von Strauss, E., Winblad, B., and Fratiglioni, L. (2004). *APOE* genotype, family history of dementia, and Alzheimer disease risk. A 6-year follow-up study. *Archives of Neurology*, **61**, 1930–1934.

Hunter, A.G.W. and Cox, D.M. (1979). Counseling problems when twins are discovered at genetic amniocentesis. *Clinical Genetics*, **16**, 34–42.

Hurst, G.P.D., Hurst, L.D., and Barrett, J.A. (1995). Meiotic drive and myotonic dystrophy. *Nature Genetics*, **10**, 132–133.

Ikeuchi, T., Igarashi, S., Takiyama, Y., et al. (1996). Non-Mendelian transmission in dentatorubral-pallidoluysian atrophy and Machado-Joseph disease: the mutant allele is preferentially transmitted in male meiosis. *American Journal of Human Genetics*, **58**, 730–733.

Iselius, L., Lindsten, J., Aurias, A., et al. (1983). The 11q:22q translocation: a collaborative study of 20 new cases and analysis of 110 families. *Human Genetics* **64**, 343–355.

Ishii, F., Fujita, H., Nagai, A., et al. (1997). Case report of rec(7)dup(7q)inv(7)(p22q22) and a review of the recombinants resulting from parental pericentric inversions on any chromosomes. *American Journal of Medical Genetics*, **73**, 290–295.

Jaber, L., Halpern, G.J., and Shohat, M. (1998). The impact of consanguinity worldwide. *Community Genetics*, **1**, 12–17.

Jalbert, P., Sele, B., and Jalbert, H. (1980). Reciprocal translocations: a way to predict the mode of imbalanced segregation by pachytene-diagram drawing. *Human Genetics* **55**, 209–222.

Jarvik, G.P., Patton, M.A., Homfray, T., and Evans, J.P. (1994). Non-Mendelian transmission in a human developmental disorder: split hand/split foot. *American Journal of Human Genetics*, **55**, 710–713.

Jeanpierre, M. (1988). A simple method for calculating risks before DNA analsyis. *Journal of Medical Genetics*, **25**, 663–668.

Johns, L.E. and Houlston, R.S. (2001). A systematic review and meta-analysis of familial colorectal cancer risk. *American Journal of Gastroenterology*, **96**, 2992–3003.

Johnson, W.F. (1980). Metabolic interference and the $+-$ heterozygote. A hypothetical form of simple inheritance which is neither dominant nor recessive. *American Journal of Human Genetics*, **32**, 374–386.

Kaiser, P. (1984). Pericentric inversions. Problems and significance for clinical genetics. *Human Genetics*, **68**, 1–47.

Kajiwara, K., Berson, E.L., and Dryja, T.P. (1994). Digenic retinitis pigmentosa due to mutations at the unlinked peripherin/*RDS* and *ROM1* loci. *Science*, **264**, 1604–1607.

Katsanis, N., Ansley, S.J., Badano, J.L. et al. (2001). Triallelic inheritance in Bardet-Biedl syndrome, a Mendelian recessive disorder. *Science*, **293**, 2256–2259.

Kaur, K., Reddy, A.B., Mukhopadhyay, A., et al. (2005). Myocilin gene implicated in primary congenital glaucoma. *Clinical Genetics*, **67**, 335–340.

Kleczkowska, A., Fryns, J.P., and Van den Bergh, H. (1987). Pericentric inversions in man: personal experience and review of the literature. *Human Genetics*, **75**, 333–338.

Köhler, J., Rupilius, B., Otto, M., Bathke, K., and Koch, M.C. (1996). Germline mosaicism in 4q35 facioscapulohumeral muscular dystrophy (FSHD1A) occurring predominantly in oogenesis. *Human Genetics*, **98**, 485–490.

Kotzot, D. and Utermann, G. (2005). Uniparental disomy (UPD) other than 15: phenotypes and bibliography updated. *American Journal of Medical Genetics*, **136A,** 287–305.

Lalouel, J.M., Morton, N.E., Maclean, C.J., and Jackson, J. (1977). Recurrence risks in complex inheritance with special regard to pyloric stenosis. *Journal of Medical Genetics*, **14,** 408–414.

Langbehn, D.R., Brinkman, R.R., Falush, D., Paulsen, J.S., and Hayden, M.R. (2004). A new model for prediction of the age of onset and penetrance for Huntingon's disease based on CAG length. *Clinical Genetics*, **65,** 267–277.

Lange, K., Westlake, J., and Spence, M.A. (1976). Extensions to pedigree analysis. II. Recurrence risk calculation under the polygenic threshold model. *Human Heredity*, **26,** 337–348.

Langford, K., Sharland, G., and Simpson, J. (2005). Relative risk of abnormal karyotype in fetuses found to have an atrioventricular septal defect (AVSD) on fetal echocardiography. *Prenatal Diagnosis*, **25,** 137–139.

Lathrop, G.M. and Lalouel, J.M. (1984). Easy calculations of lod scores and genetic risks on small computers. *American Journal of Human Genetics*, **36,** 460–465.

Lau, Y.L., Levinsky, R.J., Malcolm, S., Goodship, J., Winter, R., and Pembrey, M. (1988). Genetic prediction in X-linked agammaglobulinemia. *American Journal of Medical Genetics*, **31,** 437–448.

Leeflang, E.P., McPeek, M.S., and Arnheim, N. (1996). Analysis of meiotic segregation, using single-sperm typing: meiotic drive at the myotonic dystrophy locus. *American Journal of Human Genetics*, **59,** 896–904.

Lerer, I., Sagi, M., Ben-Neriah, Z., Wang, T., Levi, H., and Abeliovich, D. (2001). A deletion mutation in GJB6 cooperating with a GJB2 mutation in trans in non-syndromic deafness: a novel founder mutation in Ashkenazi Jews. *Human Mutation*, **18,** 460.

Liddell, M.B., Lovestone, S., and Owen, M.J. (2001). Genetic risk of Alzheimer's disease: advising relatives. *British Journal of Psychiatry*, **178,** 7–11.

Maag, U.R. and Gold, R.J.M. (1975). A simple combinatorial method for calculating genetic risks. *Clinical Genetics*, **7,** 361–367.

Madan, K. and Menko, F.H. (1992). Intrachromosomal insertions: a case report and a review. *Human Genetics*, **89,** 1–9.

Madan, K. and Nieuwint, A.W.M. (2002). Reproductive risks for paracentric inversion heterozygotes: inversion or insertion? That is the question. *American Journal of Medical Genetics*, **107,** 340–343.

Marteau, T.M., Saidi, G., Goodburn, S., Lawton, J., Michie, S., and Bobrow, M. (2000). Numbers or words? A randomized controlled trial of presenting negative results to pregnant women. *Prenatal Diagnosis*, **20,** 714–718.

Mattei, M.G., Mattei, J.F., Ayme S., and Giraud, F. (1982). X-autosome translocations: cytogenetic characteristics and their consequences. *Human Genetics*, **61,** 295–309.

McCabe, E.R.B. (2002). Hirschsprung's disease: dissecting complexity in a pathogenetic network. *Lancet*, **359,** 1169–1170.

McKusick, V.A. (1997). *Mendelian inheritance in man,* 12th ed. Johns Hopkins University Press, Baltimore.

Merryweather-Clarke, A.T., Cadet, E., Bomford, A., et al. (2003). Digenic inheritance of mutations in HAMP and HFE results in different types of hemochromatosis. *Human Molecular Genetics*, **12,** 2241–2247.

Mettler, G. and Fraser, F.C. (2000). Recurrence risk for sibs of children with "sporadic" achondroplasia. *American Journal of Medical Genetics*, **90,** 250–251.

Midro, A.T., Stengel-Rutkowski, S., and Stene, J. (1992). Experiences with risk estimates for carriers of chromosomal reciprocal translocations. *Clinical Genetics*, **41,** 113–122.

Moloney, D.M., Slaney, S.F., Oldridge, M., et al. (1996). Exclusive paternal origin of new mutations in Apert syndrome. *Nature Genetics*, **13,** 48–53.

Morissette, J., Clepet, C., Moisan, S., et al. (1998). Homozygotes carrying an autosomal dominant *TIGR* mutation do not manifest glaucoma. *Nature Genetics*, **19,** 319–321.

Morton, N.E. and Maclean, C.J. (1974). Analysis of family resemblance. III. Complex segregation of quantitative traits. *American Journal of Human Genetics*, **26,** 489–503.

Müller, B., Dechant, C., Meng, G., et al. (1992). Estimation of the male and female mutation rates in Duchenne muscular dystrophy (DMD). *Human Genetics*, **89,** 204–206.

Munier, F., Spence, M.A., Pescia, G., et al. (1992). Paternal selection favoring mutant alleles of the retinoblastoma susceptibility gene. *Human Genetics*, **89,** 508–512.

Munné, S., Dailey, T., Sultan, K.M., Grifo, J., and Cohen, J. (2000). Gamete segregation in female carriers of Robertsonian translocations. *Cytogenetics and Cell Genetics*, **90,** 303–308.

Murphy, E.A. and Mutalik, G.S. (1969). The application of Bayesian methods in genetic counseling. *Human Heredity*, **19,** 126–151.

National Advisory Council for Human Genome Research. (1994). Statement on use of DNA testing for presymptomatic identification of cancer risk. *Journal of the American Medical Association*, **271,** 785.

Noble, J. (1998). Natural history of Down's syndrome: a brief review for those involved in antenatal screening. *Journal of Medical Screening*, **5,** 172–177.

Nolin, S.L., Brown, W.T., Glicksman, A., et al., (2003). Expansion of the Fragile X CCG repeat in females with premutation or intermediate alleles. *American Journal of Human Genetics*, **72,** 454–464.

Ogino, S., Leonard, D.G.B., Rennert, H., Ewens, W.J., and Wilson, R.B. (2002). Genetic risk assessment in carrier testing for spinal muscular atrophy. *American Journal of Medical Genetics*, **110,** 301–307.

Ogino, S., Wilson, R.B., Gold, B., Hawley, P., and Grody, W.W. (2004b). Bayesian analysis for cystic fibrosis risks in prenatal and carrier screening. *Genetics in Medicine*, **6,** 439–449.

Ogino, S., Wilson, R.B., and Grody, W.W. (2004a). Bayesian risk assessment for autosomal recessive diseases: fetal echogenic bowel with one or no detectable *CFTR* mutation. *Journal of Medical Genetics*, **41,** e70.

Pai, G.S., Shields, S.M., and Houser, P.M. (1987). Segregation of inverted chromosome 13 in families ascertained through liveborn recombinant offspring. *American Journal of Medical Genetics*, **27,** 127–133.

Parmigiani, G., Berry, D., and Aguilar, O. (1998). Determining carrier probabilities for breast cancer-susceptibility genes *BRCA1* and *BRCA2*. *American Journal of Human Genetics*, **62,** 145–158.

Pauli, R.M. (1983). Dominance and homozygosity in man. *American Journal of Medical Genetics*, **16,** 455–458.

Pauli, R.M. and Motulsky, A.G. (1981). Risk counselling in autosomal dominant disorders with undetermined penetrance. *Journal of Medical Genetics*, **18,** 340–343.

Petersen, G.M., Slack, J., and Nakamura, Y. (1991). Screening guidelines and premorbid diagnosis of familial adenomatous polyposis using linkage. *Gastroenterology*, **100,** 1658–1664.

Pettenati, M.J., Rao, P.N., Phelan, M.C., et al. (1995). Paracentric inversions in humans: a review of 446 paracentric inversions with presentation of 120 new cases. *American Journal of Medical Genetics*, **55,** 171–187.

Poulton, J., Macaulay, V., and Marchington, D.R. (2003). Transmission, genetic counselling, and prenatal diagnosis of mitochondrial DNA disease. In *Genetics of mitochondrial disease* (ed. I.J.H. Holt), pp. 309–326. Oxford University Press, Oxford.

Ranen, N.G., Stine, O.C., Abbott, M.H., et al. (1995). Anticipation and instability of IT-15 (CAG)$_N$ repeats in parent–offspring pairs with Huntington disease. *American Journal of Human Genetics*, **57**, 593–602.

Rantamäki, T., Kaitila, I., Syvänen, A-C, Lukka, M., and Peltonen, L. (1999). Recurrence of Marfan syndrome as a result of parental germ-line mosaicism for an *FBN1* mutation. *American Journal of Human Genetics*, **64**, 993–1001.

Reich, T., James, J.W., and Morris, C.A. (1972). The use of multiple thresholds in determining the mode of transmission of semi-continuous traits. *Annals of Human Genetics*, **36**, 163–184.

Rose, V.M., Au, K-S., Pollom, G., Roach, S., Prashner, H.R., and Northup, H. (1999). Germ-line mosaicism in tuberous sclerosis: how common? *American Journal of Human Genetics*, **64**, 986–992.

Roux, C., Tripogney, C., Morel, F., et al. (2005). Segregation of chromosomes in sperm of Robertsonian translocation carriers. *Cytogenetic and Genome Research*, **111**, 291–296.

Ryan, S.G., Chance, P.F., Zou, C., Spinner, N.B., Golden, J.A., and Smietana, S. (1997). Epilepsy and mental retardation limited to females: an X-linked dominant disorder with male sparing. *Nature Genetics*, **17**, 92–95.

Savage, D.B., Agostini, M., Barrosa, I., et al. (2002). Digenic inheritance of severe insulin resistance in a human pedigree. *Nature Genetics*, **31**, 379–384.

Schinzel, A. (1994). *Human cytogenetics database*. Oxford University Press, Oxford.

Schinzel, A. (2001). *Catalogue of unbalanced chromosome aberrations in man*, 2nd ed. Walter de Gruyter, Berlin.

Schmidt, M. and Du Sart, D. (1992). Functional disomies of the X chromosome influence the cell selection and hence the X inactivation pattern in females with balanced X-autosome translocations: a review of 122 cases. *American Journal of Medical Genetics*, **42**, 161–169.

Schmidt, S., Becher, H., and Chang-Claude, J. (1998). Breast cancer risk assessment: use of complete pedigree information and the effect of misspecified ages at diagnosis of affected relatives. *Human Genetics*, **102**, 348–356.

Schorderet, D.F., Friedman, C., and Disteche, C.M. (1991). Pericentric inversion of the X chromosome: presentation of a case and review of the literature. *Annals de Génétique*, **34**, 98–103.

Scotet, V., De Braekeleer, M., Audrézet, M-P., et al. (2002). Prenatal detection of cystic fibrosis by ultrasonography: a retrospective study of more than 346,000 pregnancies. *Journal of Medical Genetics*, **39**, 443–448.

Seshadri, S., Drachman, D.A., and Lippa, C.F. (1995). Apolipoprotein E ε4 allele and the lifetime risk of Alzheimer's disease. *Archives of Neurology*, **52**, 1074–1079.

Shaw, A.M., Bernetson, R.A., Phillips, M.F., Harper, P.S., and Harley, H.G. (1995). Evidence for meiotic drive at the myotonic dystrophy locus. *Journal of Medical Genetics*, **32**, 145.

Sherman, S.L., Iselius, L., Gallano, P., et al. (1986). Segregation analysis of balanced pericentric inversions in pedigree data. *Clinical Genetics*, **30**, 87–94.

Sibert, J.R., Harper, P.S., Thompson, R.J., and Newcombe, R.G. (1979). Carrier detection in Duchenne muscular dystrophy. *Archives of Disease in Childhood*, **54**, 534–537.

Silverstein, S., Lerer, I., Sagi, M., et al. (2002). Uniparental disomy in fetuses diagnosed with balanced translocations: risk estimate. *Prenatal Diagnosis*, **22**, 649–651.

Sippel, K.C., Fraioli, R.E., Smith, G.D., et al. (1998). Frequency of somatic and germ-line mosaicism in retinoblastoma: implications for genetic counselling. *American Journal of Human Genetics*, **62**, 610–619.

Smith, C. (1971). Recurrrence risks for multifactorial inheritance. *American Journal of Human Genetics*, **23**, 578–588.

Smith, C. (1972). Computer programme to estimate recurrence risks for multifactorial familial disease. *British Medical Journal*, **1**, 495–497.

Stene, J. (1970a). Statistical inference on segregation ratios for D/G translocations when the families are ascertained in different ways. *Annals of Human Genetics*, **34**, 93–115.

Stene, J. (1970b). A statistical segregation analysis of (21q22q) translocations. *Human Heredity*, **20**, 465–472.

Stene, J. and Stengel-Rutkowski, S. (1988). Genetic risks of familial reciprocal and Robertsonian translocation carriers. In *The cytogenetics of mammalian autosomal rearrangements* (ed. A. Daniel), pp. 3–72. Alan R Liss, New York.

Stengel-Rutkowski, S., Stene, J., and Gallano, P. (1988). Risk estimates in balanced parental reciprocal translocations. Analysis of 1120 pedigrees. *Monographie des Annales de Génétique*. Expansion Scientifique Française, Paris.

Stengel-Rutkowski, S., Warkotsch, A., Schimanek, P., and Stene, J. (1984). Familial Wolf's syndrome with a hidden 4p deletion by translocation of an 8p segment. Unbalanced inheritance from a maternal translocation (4;8)(p15.3;p22). Case report, review and risk estimates. *Clinical Genetics*, **25**, 500–521.

Sutherland, G.R., Callen, D.F., and Gardner, R.J.M. (1995). Paracentric inversions do not normally generate monocentric recombinant chromosomes. *American Journal of Medical Genetics*, **59**, 390.

Sutherland, G.R., Gardiner, A.J., and Carter, R.F. (1976). Familial pericentric inversion of chromosome 19, inv(19)(p13q13) with a note on genetic counselling of pericentric inversion carriers. *Clinical Genetics*, **10**, 54–59.

Takiyama, Y., Sakoe, K., Amaike, M., et al. (1999). Single sperm analysis of the CAG repeats in the gene for dentatorubral-pallidoluysian atrophy (DRPLA): the instability of the CAG repeats in the *DRPLA* gene is prominent among the CAG repeat diseases. *Human Molecular Genetics*, **8**, 453–457.

Therman, E. and Kuhn, E.M. (1981). Mitotic crossing-over and segregation in man. *Human Genetics*, **59**, 93–100.

Therman, E., Laxova, R., and Susman, B. (1990). The critical region on the human Xq. *Human Genetics*, **85**, 455–461.

Thomas, G.H. (1996). High male:female ratio of germ-line mutations: an alternative explanation for postulated genetic lethality in males in X-linked dominant disorders. *American Journal of Human Genetics*, **58**, 1364–1368.

Tuchman, M., Matsudo, I., Munnich, A., Malcolm, S., Strautnieks, S., and Briede, T. (1995). Proportions of spontaneous mutations in males and females with ornithine transcarbamylase deficiency. *American Journal of Medical Genetics*, **55**, 67–70.

Twigg, S.R.F., Kan, R., Babbs, C., et al. (2004). Mutations of ephrin-B1 (*EFNB1*), a marker of tissue boundary formation, cause craniofrontonasal syndrome. *Proceedings of the National Academy of Science*, **101**, 8652–8657.

Van der Maarel, S.M. and Frants, R.R. (2005). The D4Z4 repeat-mediated pathogenesis of facioscapulohumeral muscular dystrophy. *American Journal of Human Genetics*, **76**, 375–386.

Van der Meulen, M.A., van der Meulen, M.J.P., and te Meerman, G.J. (1995). Recurrence risk for germinal mosaics revisited. *Journal of Medical Genetics*, **32**, 102–105.

Van Essen, A.J., Abbs, S., Barget, M., et al. (1992). Parental origin and germline mosaicism of deletions and duplications of the dystrophin gene: a European study. *Human Genetics*, **88**, 249–257.

Van Hemel, J.O. and Eussen, H.J. (2000). Interchromosomal insertions. Identification of five cases and a review. *Human Genetics*, **107**, 415–432.

Vekemans, M. and Morichon-Delvallez, N. (1990). Duplication of the long arm of chromosome 13 secondary to a recombination in a maternal intrachromosomal insertion (shift). *Prenatal Diagnosis*, **10,** 787–794.

White, S.L., Collins, V.R., Wolfe, R., et al. (1999). Genetic counseling and prenatal diagnosis for the mitochondrial DNA mutations at nucleotide 8993. *American Journal of Human Genetics*, **65,** 474–482.

Wieland, I., Jakubiczka, S., Muschke, P., et al. (2004). Mutations of the *Ephrin-B1* gene cause craniofrontonasal syndrome. *American Journal of Human Genetics*, **74,** 1209–1215.

Winter, R.M. (1985). The estimation of recurrence risks in monogenic disorders using flanking marker loci. *Journal of Medical Genetics*, **22,** 12–15.

Wordsworth, P. and Brown, M. (1997). Rheumatoid arthritis and allied inflammatory arthropathies. In *Principles and practice of medical genetics*, 3rd ed. (eds D.L. Rimoin, J.M. Connor, and R. Pyeritz), pp. 2751–2772. Churchill Livingstone, New York.

Zheng, Q.Y., Yan, D., Ouyang, X.M., et al. (2005). Digenic inheritance of deafness caused by mutations in genes encoding cadherin 23 and protocadherin 15 in mice and humans. *Human Molecular Genetics*, **14,** 103–111.

Zlotogora, J. (1997). Dominance and homozygosity. *American Journal of Medical Genetics*, **68,** 412–416.

Zunc, E., Abeliovich, D., Halpern, G.J., Magal, N., and Shohat, M. (2004). Myotonic dystrophy—no evidence for preferential transmission of the mutated allele: a prenatal analysis. *American Journal of Medical Genetics*, **127A,** 50–53.

Appendix A1: Ultrasound and Prenatal Diagnosis

Ultrasonography is now undertaken routinely for the detection of fetal abnormalities during the second trimester of pregnancy. This can often reveal the presence of an abnormality that raises concern that the fetus has a more serious underlying diagnosis. The finding may take the form of a "hard" malformation such as an atrioventricular septal defect (AVSD) or duodenal atresia. Alternatively, it may represent one of a number of "soft" markers such as nuchal translucency or hyperechogenic bowel. These findings are known to convey increased risks for chromosome disorders such as Down syndrome and, in the case of hyperechogenic bowel, for cystic fibrosis. However, calculation of the precise risk can prove to be very difficult.

To determine the risk, it is necessary to have background information on the strength of the association between the ultrasound finding and the suspected underlying diagnosis. This may take one of two forms. Information may be available from the literature indicating the incidence of the particular finding in the relevant syndrome, (e.g., 5% of babies with Down syndrome have duodenal atresia), or the proportion of babies with a particular finding who have a specific underlying syndrome may be known (e.g., 50% of babies with an AVSD have Down syndrome). In both of these situations it is crucial to take prior probabilities into account. This is illustrated in the following examples.

Example 1: Duodenal Atresia and Down Syndrome

Routine fetal anomaly ultrasound scanning reveals the presence of duodenal atresia with no other obvious abnormality. The mother is aged 25 years. It is known that the incidence of duodenal atresia in babies with Down syndrome is 1 in 20, in contrast to the incidence of approximately 1 in 5000 in babies not affected with Down syndrome. This does not mean that the odds that the fetus has Down syndrome are 250 to 1.

219

Table A1.1. (see Example 1).

Probability	Fetus Is Affected	Fetus Is Not Affected
Prior	1/1500	≈ 1
Conditional		
Duodenal atresia	1/20	1/5000
Joint	1/30,000	1/5000

Posterior probability that the fetus is affected equals 1/30,000/(1/30,000 + 1/5000) equals 1/7

It represents only the conditional probability based on the ultrasound findings. To determine the correct probability, the prior probability that the fetus is affected with Down syndrome has to be taken into account. This is dependent upon the mother's age. The correct probability that the fetus is affected can be determined by a simple Bayesian calculation, as shown in Table A1.1. This yields an overall risk of 1 in 7. Note that for an older mother of age 40 years, for whom the prior probability is approximately 1 in 100, the risk is much higher, i.e., 5/7, as shown in Table A1.2.

Example 2: Atrioventricular Septal Defect and Down Syndrome

In this example a fetus is found on routine ultrasonography to have an AVSD. The mother is aged 30 years. At the prenatal diagnostic center where this test was undertaken, it has been shown in a large study sample that approximately 50% of all fetuses with an AVSD have Down syndrome. However, this does not mean that the mother can be counseled that there is a risk of 1 in 2 that her unborn baby is affected, as once again, this does not take into account the prior risk. To provide her with a more correct estimate, it is necessary to calculate in the study sample the relative risk that the fetus is affected based on comparison of the observed and expected numbers of affected babies, taking into account the prior age-related maternal risks. In this way, a conditional probability can be obtained and then incorporated into a Bayesian calculation. In one such study a relative risk of 107 was obtained (Langford et al., 2005).

Table A1.2. (see Example 1).

Probability	Fetus Is Affected	Fetus Is Not Affected
Prior	1/100	≈ 1
Conditional		
Duodenal atresia	1/20	1/5000
Joint	1/2000	1/5000

Posterior probability that the fetus is affected equals 1/2000/(1/2000 + 1/5000) equals 5/7

Table A1.3. (see Example 2).

Probability	Fetus Is Affected	Fetus Is Not Affected
Prior	1/1000	≈ 1
Conditional		
AVSD	107	1
Joint	107/1000	1

Posterior probability that the fetus is affected equals 107/1000/(107/1000 + 1) equals 0.096

AVSD, atrioventricular septal defect.

Alternatively, reference can be made to epidemiological surveys to determine the incidence of AVSD in babies with Down syndrome. These indicate an overall incidence of approximately 1 in 5 (Noble, 1998).

The probability that the fetus is affected is then calculated as shown in Tables A1.3 and A1.4, taking into account the prior probability based on the mother's age and the observed incidence of Down syndrome at the relevant gestation. For a 30-year-old woman this is approximately 1 in 1000. The calculation in Table A1.3, using a conditional probability of 107 to 1 as derived in the prenatal study, gives a posterior probability of 0.096 or roughly 1 in 10 that the fetus is affected. Table A1.4, using conditional probabilities of 1 in 5 and 1 in 1000, gives a posterior probability of 1 in 6 that the fetus is affected. The fact that the posterior probabilities obtained using these two approaches are not the same reflects the difference in the ways in which the conditional probabilities were derived and that they were derived from different data.

Example 3: Hyperechogenic Bowel and Cystic Fibrosis

Hyperechogenic bowel, defined as echogenicity equal to or greater than that of surrounding bone, can occur as a normal variant. It can also be a manifestation of an important underlying diagnosis such as congenital infection, Down syndrome,

Table A1.4. AVSD and Down Syndrome

Probability	Fetus Is Affected	Fetus Is Not Affected
Prior	1/1000	≈ 1
Conditional		
AVSD	1/5	1/1000
Joint	1/5000	1/1000

Posterior probability that the fetus is affected equals 1/5000/(1/5000 + 1/1000) equals 1/6

AVSD, atrioventricular septal defect.

Table A1.5. (see Example 3).

Probability	Fetus Is Affected	Fetus Is Not Affected
Prior (population frequency)	1/2500	≈ 1
Conditional		
Hyperechogenic bowel	0.11	0.0004
One mutation detected	0.18	0.04 × 0.9*
Joint	0.0000079	0.000144

Posterior probability that the fetus is affected equals 0.0000079/(0.0000079 + 0.000144) equals 0.052

*This conditional probability is derived by multiplying the frequency of carriers in the general population (1 in 25 = 0.04) by the proportion of carriers in whom a mutation can be identified (0.9).

or cystic fibrosis. In this example, mutation analysis is undertaken following placental biopsy, and a single pathogenic cystic fibrosis mutation is identified. What is the probability that the fetus is affected? The molecular test used for the analysis detects 90% of all mutations, and the local incidence of cystic fibrosis is 1 in 2500.

To answer this question, it is necessary to know either the proportion of babies with cystic fibrosis who have hyperechogenic bowel or the proportion of babies with hyperechogenic bowel who have cystic fibrosis. Data from the literature indicate that the incidence of hyperechogenic bowel in fetuses with and without cystic fibrosis is approximately 11% and 0.04%, respectively (Scotet et al., 2002), although widely differing figures have been obtained in different studies. The proportion of babies with hyperechogenic bowel who have cystic fibrosis will depend on the incidence of cystic fibrosis in the relevant population; a figure of 2%–3% is usually quoted for populations with a high frequency (Bosco et al., 1999). Ideally, in practice, local data should be used to take into account both the frequency of cystic fibrosis in the relevant population and local practice relating to the definition and detection of bowel hyperechogenicity.

The probability that the fetus is affected can be calculated as shown in Tables A1.5 and A1.6. Table A1.5 uses conditional probabilities based on the incidence of bowel hyperechogenicity in babies with and without cystic fibrosis and the proportions of affected/unaffected babies in whom only one mutation can be detected. These parameters are probably independent, although there is some evidence that

Table A1.6. (see Example 3).

Probability	Fetus Is Affected	Fetus Is Not Affected
Prior (hyperechogenic bowel)	1/50	49/50
Conditional		
One mutation detected	0.18	0.04 × 0.9
Joint	0.0036	0.03528

Posterior probability that the fetus is affected equals 0.0036/(0.0036 + 0.03528) equals 0.0925

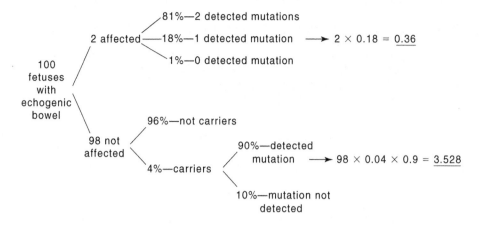

Proportion of fetuses with 1 detected mutation which are affected

$$= \frac{0.36}{0.36 + 3.528} = 0.093$$

Figure A1.1. A flow diagram showing how the risk for cystic fibrosis can be calculated in a fetus with hyperechogenic bowel and a single cystic fibrosis mutation.

bowel hyperechogenicity may be slightly more common in babies with one mutation than in those with none (Scotet et al., 2002). This method gives a risk of roughly 1 in 20. Table A1.6 uses prior probabilities based on the observed incidence of cystic fibrosis in babies with bowel hyperechogenicity and yields a risk of roughly 1 in 11. These methods give different results because the data used have been obtained from different sources. In practice, these figures indicate the range in which the true risk is likely to fall and may enable the prospective parents to make a decision about how they wish to proceed.

Cystic fibrosis mutation analysis in pregnancies with bowel hyperechogenicity can generate some very difficult risk calculations. Various approaches to how these can be resolved have been considered by Hodge et al. (1999) and by Ogino et al. (2004a, b). Those with an intense dislike of Bayesian analysis might prefer the flow diagram approach used by Bosco et al. (1999). This is illustrated in Figure A1.1. Essentially, it is very similar to the Bayesian approach shown in Table A1.6.

Appendix A2: Overlapping Normal Distributions

Overlapping normal distributions are often used in genetic counseling. Examples include the maternal serum alpha fetoprotein levels in healthy babies and those with open neural tube defects, and serum creatine kinase levels in healthy controls and obligatory carriers of DMD. Knowledge of the statistical parameters (mean and standard deviation) of each of the overlapping normal curves can be used to derive conditional probabilities for the result obtained in a particular consultand. These conditional probabilities must then be incorporated into a Bayesian calculation taking into account prior probabilities. This is because the overlapping curves, which will have been constructed using results from small numbers of controls and carriers, grossly distort the true population picture, which will contain a massive excess of healthy controls with the carrier curve being minute in comparison.

The normal (Gaussian) distribution is a symmetrical bell-shaped curve distributed about a mean. The spread of the distribution about the mean is determined by the standard deviation, which is located on the point of the curve at which it changes from a convex to a concave shape. Approximately 68%, 95%, and 99.7% of observations fall within the mean ± 1, 2, and 3 standard deviations, respectively. In theory, the normal distribution curve extends to infinity in both directions, so that strictly speaking, human characteristics such as height and IQ could not conform exactly to a normal distribution. However, in practice, many human measurements correspond very closely to a normal distribution either directly or following transformation by techniques such as conversion to logarithmic values.

The standard normal deviate relates to a standardized normal distribution with a mean of 0 and standard deviation of 1. By converting an observation from a normal distribution to a standard normal deviate, it is possible to use tables of standard normal variables for probability calculations. Any value (X) in a normal distribution can be transformed to a standard normal deviate (Z) by subtracting the mean (M) and then dividing by the standard deviation (SD), i.e., $Z = (X - M)/SD$. One of the many potential applications of standard normal deviates is that they can be used to derive conditional probabilities that a particular result will fall in different overlapping normal distributions. This is illustrated by the following example.

A woman with a prior probability of 0.33 for being a carrier of DMD has had serum creatine kinase (CK) measured on three occasions resulting in a mean log value of 1.9. Distributions for serum CK have been obtained for healthy controls and for obligatory carriers. When plotted using log CK values, two overlapping curves are obtained, each of which approximates to the normal distribution, with mean and standard deviations of 1.69 and 0.15 for the controls and 2.18 and 0.35 for the obligatory carriers.

Conditional probabilities for the consultand being a carrier or not a carrier are calculated as follows.

The standard normal deviate $(X - M)/SD$ is calculated for each distribution.

$$\text{Controls: } Z1 = \frac{1.9 - 1.69}{0.15} = 1.4$$

$$\text{Carriers: } Z2 = \frac{1.9 - 2.18}{0.35} = -0.8$$

Using these values, the height or probability density (P) is calculated for each normal curve from the function

$$\frac{1}{SD\sqrt{(2\pi)} \times \exp(Z^2/2)}$$

$$\text{Controls: } P1 = \frac{1}{0.15 \times 2.5066 \times \exp 0.98} = 0.9982$$

$$\text{Carriers: } P2 = \frac{1}{0.35 \times 2.5066 \times \exp 0.32} = 0.8277$$

Finally, these conditional probabilities are multiplied by the prior probabilities (Table A2.1).

Table A2.1.

Probability	Carrier	Not a Carrier
Prior	0.333	0.667
Conditional	0.8277	0.9982
Joint	0.2756	0.6658

This gives a posterior probability of

$$\frac{0.2756}{0.2756 + 0.6658} = 0.29$$

that the consultant is a carrier.

In practice, it is customary to calculate conditional probabilities for several CK values and then convert these to likelihood ratios that can be plotted to construct a graph of odds versus CK level. This enables an odds ratio to be read off quickly for any CK value (Dennis and Carter, 1978; Sibert et al., 1979).

Appendix A3: Length of Prometaphase Chromosome Segments

As indicated in Chapter 9, one approach to predicting the likely viability of chromosome imbalance that could be generated by malsegregation of a balanced parental chromosome rearrangement involves direct measurement of the extent of imbalance. Toward this end, the sizes of prometaphase chromosomes and their segments at the 750 band level have been published by Daniel (1985) and are reproduced in Tables A3.1 and A3.2. The values in Table A3.2 for each band relate to the distance from the interband between that band and the next band to the telomere, so that a mid-band breakpoint value can be obtained by using the average of the values indicated for each band and the band above. The length of an interstitial segment can be calculated by subtracting the value at the distal breakpoint from that indicated for the proximal breakpoint.

Table A3.1. Length of Prometaphase Chromosomes Expressed as a Percentage of the Total Haploid Autosome Length

Chromosome	Short Arm	Long Arm	Total Length
1	4.61	4.63	9.24
2	3.27	5.47	8.75
3	3.27	3.74	7.01
4	1.71	4.99	6.70
5	1.61	4.68	6.29
6	2.33	3.97	6.30
7	2.06	3.50	5.55
8	1.59	3.33	4.92
9	1.60	3.22	4.81
10	1.48	3.24	4.72
11	1.62	2.99	4.60
12	1.30	3.57	4.86
13	—	3.26	3.26
14	—	3.24	3.24
15	—	3.06	3.06
16	1.23	1.92	3.15
17	0.96	2.50	3.46
18	0.70	1.90	2.60
19	1.11	1.36	2.47
20	0.93	1.35	2.28
21	—	1.22	1.22
22	—	1.47	1.47
X	2.06	3.27	5.32
Y	0.37	1.44	1.82

Source: Adapted with permission from Daniel, A (1985). The size of prometaphase chromosome segments. *Clinical Genetics*. **28**, 216–224. © Blackwell Publishing Ltd., Oxford.

Table A3.2. Prometaphase Chromosome Segment Sizes Expressed as a Percentage of the Total Haploid Autosome Length

Chromosome Band (Short Arm)	Distance of Interband Border to Telomere	Chromosome Band (Long Arm)	Distance of Interband Border to Telomere
1p11	4.47	1q11	—
1p12	4.38	1q12	4.04
1p13.1	4.29	1q21.1	3.84
1p13.2	4.15	1q21.2	3.75
1p13.3	3.92	1q21.3	3.56
1p21.1	—	1q22	3.47
1p21.3	3.64	1q23.1	3.19
1p22.1	3.41	1q23.2	3.03
1p22.2	3.27	1q23.3	2.87
1p22.3	3.09	1q24.1	2.79
1p31.1	2.67	1q24.2	2.71
1p31.2	2.58	1q24.3	2.63
1p31.3	2.44	1q25.1	2.46
1p32.1	2.26	1q25.2	2.38
1p32.2	2.08	1q25.3	2.14
1p32.3	1.89	1q31.1	2.02
1p33	1.80	1q31.2	1.94
1p34.1	1.52	1q31.3	1.82
1p34.2	1.38	1q32.1	1.45
1p34.3	1.20	1q32.2	1.37
1p35.1	1.11	1q32.3	1.29
1p35.2	1.01	1q41	1.09
1p35.3	0.92	1q42.11	1.01
1p36.11	0.83	1q42.12	0.93
1p36.12	0.74	1q42.13	0.69
1p36.13	0.51	1q42.2	0.61
1p36.21	0.42	1q42.3	0.44
1p36.22	0.32	1q43	0.24
1p36.23	—	1q44	0.00
1p36.33	0.00		
2p11.1	3.11	2q11.1	5.42
2p11.2	2.85	2q11.2	5.20
2p12	2.58	2q12	4.98
2p13	2.32	2q13	4.70
2p14	2.16	2q14.1	4.54
2p15	2.03	2q14.2	4.38
2p16.1	1.93	2q14.3	4.21
2p16.2	1.90	2q21.1	3.94
2p16.3	1.73	2q21.2	3.88
2p21	1.50	2q21.3	3.83
2p22.1	1.41	2q22	3.61
2p22.2	1.37	2q23.1	3.56
2p22.3	1.18	2q23.2	3.45
2p23.1	1.08	2q23.3	3.28
2p23.2	1.05	2q24.1	3.12
2p23.3	0.92	2q24.2	2.95
2p24.1	0.75	2q24.3	2.74
2p24.2	0.69	2q31.1	2.41
2p24.3	0.49	2q31.2	2.30
2p25.1	0.29	2q31.3	2.24
2p25.2	0.16	2q32.1	2.02
2p25.3	0.00	2q32.2	1.97
		2q32.3	1.81

(continued)

Chromosome Band (Short Arm)	Distance of Interband Border to Telomere	Chromosome Band (Long Arm)	Distance of Interband Border to Telomere
		2q33.1	1.48
		2q33.2	1.42
		2q33.3	1.31
		2q34	1.09
		2q35	0.88
		2q36.1	0.71
		2q36.2	0.66
		2q36.3	0.49
		2q37.1	0.33
		2q37.2	0.27
		2q37.3	0.00
3p11	—	3q11	3.52
3p12	2.85	3q12	3.37
3p13	2.65	3q13.11	3.25
3p14.1	2.55	3q13.12	—
3p14.2	2.42	3q13.2	2.96
3p14.3	2.29	3q13.31	2.88
3p21.1	—	3q13.32	2.84
3p21.2	2.03	3q13.33	2.77
3p21.31	1.57	3q21	2.32
3p21.32	1.47	3q22.1	2.21
3p21.33	1.31	3q22.2	2.09
3p22	1.11	3q22.3	2.02
3p23	0.98	3q23	1.83
3p24.1	0.88	3q24	1.65
3p24.2	0.85	3q25.1	1.46
3p24.3	0.62	3q25.2	1.35
3p25.1	0.43	3q25.3	1.23
3p25.2	0.36	3q26.1	1.05
3p25.3	0.20	3q26.2	0.94
3p26.1	0.13	3q26.31	0.82
3p26.2	0.07	3q26.32	0.75
3p26.3	0.00	3q26.33	0.67
		3q27	0.37
		3q28	0.22
		3q29	0.00
4p11	1.63	4q11	4.64
4p12	1.54	4q12	4.44
4p13	1.40	4q13.1	4.39
4p14	1.21	4q13.2	4.19
4p15.1	0.99	4q13.3	4.04
4p15.2	0.86	4q21.1	3.97
4p15.31	0.70	4q21.21	3.92
4p15.32	0.58	4q21.22	3.84
4p15.33	0.45	4q21.23	3.64
4p16.1	0.33	4q21.3	3.39
4p16.2	0.15	4q22	3.19
4p16.3	0.00	4q23	2.99
		4q24	2.86
		4q25	2.72
		4q26	2.55
		4q27	2.40
		4q28.1	2.25
		4q28.2	2.15
		4q28.3	1.80

Chromosome Band (Short Arm)	Distance of Interband Border to Telomere	Chromosome Band (Long Arm)	Distance of Interband Border to Telomere
		4q31.1	1.65
		4q31.21	1.50
		4q31.22	1.40
		4q31.23	1.30
		4q31.3	1.20
		4q32.11	1.05
		4q32.2	0.95
		4q32.3	0.75
		4q33	0.70
		4q34.1	0.55
		4q34.2	0.50
		4q34.3	0.40
		4q35.1	0.15
		4q35.2	0.00
5p11	1.51	5q11.1	4.40
5p12	1.40	5q11.2	4.21
5p13.1	1.30	5q12	4.02
5p13.2	1.18	5q13.1	3.84
5p13.3	0.92	5q13.2	3.74
5p14	0.63	5q13.3	3.60
5p15.1	0.48	5q14.1	3.51
5p15.2	0.37	5q14.2	3.32
5p15.31	0.26	5q14.3	3.04
5p15.32	0.18	5q15	2.86
5p15.33	0.00	5q21.1	2.76
		5q21.2	2.67
		5q21.3	2.53
		5q22	2.29
		5q23.1	2.11
		5q23.2	1.97
		5q23.3	1.83
		5q31.1	1.59
		5q31.2	1.50
		5q31.3	1.31
		5q32	1.12
		5q33.1	0.98
		5q33.2	0.84
		5q33.3	0.70
		5q34	0.52
		5q35.1	0.33
		5q35.2	0.23
		5q35.3	0.00
6p11	2.31	6q11	3.89
6p12.1	2.10	6q12	3.61
6p12.2	2.07	6q13	3.49
6p12.3	1.86	6q14.1	3.34
6p21.1	1.79	6q14.2	3.30
6p21.2	1.42	6q14.3	3.14
6p21.3	1.03	6q15	2.94
6p22.1	0.89	6q16.1	2.74
6p22.2	0.79	6q16.2	2.66
6p22.3	0.58	6q16.3	2.50
6p23	0.47	6q21	2.14
6p24.1	0.40	6q22.1	2.03
6p24.2	0.37	6q22.2	1.95

(continued)

Chromosome Band (Short Arm)	Distance of Interband Border to Telomere	Chromosome Band (Long Arm)	Distance of Interband Border to Telomere
6p24.3	0.26	6q22.31	1.79
6p25	0.00	6q22.32	1.67
		6q22.33	1.47
		6q23.1	1.27
		6q23.2	1.11
		6q23.3	1.03
		6q24	0.91
		6q25.1	0.72
		6q25.2	0.60
		6q25.3	0.32
		6q26	0.20
		6q27	0.00
7p11.1	2.02	7q11.1	3.47
7p11.2	1.88	7q11.21	3.22
7p12.1	1.81	7q11.22	3.12
7p12.2	1.77	7q11.23	2.87
7p12.3	1.71	7q21.11	2.66
7p13	1.44	7q21.12	2.56
7p14.1	1.32	7q21.13	2.45
7p14.2	1.26	7q21.2	2.35
7p14.3	1.15	7q21.3	2.24
7p15.1	0.99	7q22.1	1.89
7p15.2	0.89	7q22.2	1.79
7p15.3	0.68	7q22.3	1.68
7p21	0.39	7q31.1	1.58
7p22	0.00	7q31.2	1.47
		7q31.31	1.33
		7q31.32	1.26
		7q31.33	1.16
		7q32	0.88
		7q33	0.74
		7q34	0.60
		7q35	0.42
		7q36.1	0.28
		7q36.2	0.21
		7q36.3	0.00
8p11.1	1.50	8q11.1	3.30
8p11.21	1.37	8q11.21	3.16
8p11.22	1.34	8q11.22	3.03
8p11.23	1.24	8q11.23	2.83
8p12	1.07	8q12.1	2.73
8p21.1	0.89	8q12.2	2.66
8p21.2	0.83	8q12.3	2.56
8p21.3	0.65	8q13.1	2.46
8p22	0.62	8q13.2	2.40
8p23.1	0.25	8q13.3	2.23
8p23.2	0.13	8q21.11	2.10
8p23.3	0.00	8q21.12	2.07
		8q21.13	1.93
		8q21.2	1.83
		8q21.3	1.67
		8q22.1	1.50
		8q22.2	1.43
		8q22.3	1.23

Chromosome Band (Short Arm)	Distance of Interband Border to Telomere	Chromosome Band (Long Arm)	Distance of Interband Border to Telomere
		8q23.1	—
		8q23.3	0.93
		8q24.11	0.80
		8q24.12	0.73
		8q24.13	0.60
		8q24.21	0.50
		8q24.22	0.40
		8q24.23	0.30
		8q24.3	0.00
9p11.1	1.55	9q11	—
9p11.2	1.44	9q12	2.65
9p12	1.30	9q13	2.54
9p13.1	1.23	9q21.11	2.47
9p13.2	1.15	9q21.12	2.39
9p13.3	0.98	9q21.13	2.28
9p21.1	0.83	9q21.2	2.17
9p21.2	0.78	9q21.31	2.04
9p21.3	0.69	9q21.32	1.91
9p22.1	0.59	9q21.33	1.80
9p22.2	0.51	9q22.1	1.64
9p22.3	0.43	9q22.2	1.59
9p23	0.29	9q22.31	1.48
9p24	0.00	9q22.32	1.43
		9q22.33	1.27
		9q31.1	1.14
		9q31.2	1.03
		9q31.3	0.98
		9q32	0.82
		9q33.1	0.69
		9q33.2	0.61
		9q33.3	0.53
		9q34.11	0.35
		9q34.12	0.32
		9q34.13	0.24
		9q34.2	0.21
		9q34.3	0.00
10p11.1	1.38	10q11.1	3.11
10p11.21	1.24	10q11.21	2.95
10p11.22	1.17	10q11.22	2.92
10p11.23	1.02	10q11.23	2.75
10p12.1	—	10q21.1	2.56
10p12.33	0.67	10q21.2	2.50
10p13	0.47	10q21.3	2.33
10p14	0.33	10q22.1	2.07
10p15.1	0.21	10q22.2	1.98
10p15.2	0.15	10q22.3	1.81
10p15.3	0.00	10q23.1	1.69
		10q23.2	1.62
		10q23.31	1.49
		10q23.32	1.36
		10q23.33	1.26
		10q24	1.04
		10q25.1	0.91
		10q25.2	0.81
		10q25.3	0.71

(continued)

Chromosome Band (Short Arm)	Distance of Interband Border to Telomere	Chromosome Band (Long Arm)	Distance of Interband Border to Telomere
		10q26.11	0.62
		10q26.12	0.52
		10q26.13	0.32
		10q26.2	0.23
		10q26.3	0.00
11p11.11	1.54	11q11	2.93
11p11.12	1.41	11q12.1	2.78
11p11.2	1.25	11q12.2	2.60
11p12	1.05	11q12.3	2.54
11p13	0.91	11q13.1	2.39
11p14	0.66	11q13.2	2.33
11p15.1	0.57	11q13.3	2.09
11p15.2	0.47	11q13.4	1.97
11p15.3	0.39	11q13.5	1.85
11p15.4	0.28	11q14.1	1.70
11p15.5	0.00	11q14.2	1.62
		11q14.3	1.47
		11q21	1.38
		11q22.1	1.23
		11q22.2	1.14
		11q22.3	0.99
		11q23.1	0.90
		11q23.2	0.81
		11q23.3	0.57
		11q24.1	0.42
		11q24.2	0.33
		11q24.3	0.18
		11q25	0.00
12p11.1	1.22	12q11	3.53
12p11.21	1.04	12q12	3.25
12p11.22	0.98	12q13.11	3.14
12p11.23	0.91	12q13.12	3.03
12p12	0.61	12q13.13	2.79
12p13.1	0.49	12q13.2	2.68
12p13.2	0.39	12q13.3	2.57
12p13.31	0.21	12q14	2.36
12p13.32	0.14	12q15	2.18
12p13.33	0.00	12q21.1	2.04
		12q21.2	1.90
		12q21.3	1.54
		12q22	1.39
		12q23.1	1.25
		12q23.2	1.18
		12q23.3	1.07
		12q24.1	0.75
		12q24.2	0.61
		12q24.31	0.43
		12q24.32	0.32
		12q24.33	0.00
13p11		13q11	3.20
13p12		13q12.11	3.06
13p13		13q12.12	3.03
		13q12.13	2.93
		13q12.2	2.87

Chromosome Band (Short Arm)	Distance of Interband Border to Telomere	Chromosome Band (Long Arm)	Distance of Interband Border to Telomere
		13q12.3	2.74
		13q13.1	2.67
		13q13.2	2.61
		13q13.3	2.45
		13q14.11	2.25
		13q14.12	2.22
		13q14.13	2.12
		13q14.2	2.02
		13q14.3	1.89
		13q21.11	1.76
		13q21.2	1.63
		13q21.31	1.53
		13q21.32	1.43
		13q21.33	1.30
		13q22.1	1.21
		13q22.2	1.17
		13q22.3	1.08
		13q31.1	0.88
		13q31.2	0.85
		13q31.3	0.72
		13q32.1	0.59
		13q32.2	0.55
		13q32.3	0.39
		13q33	0.23
		13q34	0.00
14p11		14q11.1	3.08
14p12		14q11.2	2.85
14p13		14q12	2.69
		14q13.1	2.59
		14q13.2	2.53
		14q13.3	2.43
		14q21.1	2.27
		14q21.2	2.24
		14q21.3	2.11
		14q22.1	1.91
		14q22.2	1.85
		14q22.3	1.78
		14q23.1	1.65
		14q23.2	1.56
		14q23.3	1.49
		14q24.1	1.36
		14q24.2	1.30
		14q24.3	0.97
		14q31	0.68
		14q32.1	0.49
		14q32.2	0.42
		14q32.31	0.32
		14q32.32	0.26
		14q32.33	0.00
15p11		15q11.1	3.00
15p12		15q11.2	2.79
15p13		15q12	2.66
		15q13.1	2.54
		15q13.2	2.49

(*continued*)

Chromosome Band (Short Arm)	Distance of Interband Border to Telomere	Chromosome Band (Long Arm)	Distance of Interband Border to Telomere
		15q13.3	2.30
		15q14	2.14
		15q15.1	1.99
		15q15.2	1.96
		15q15.3	1.84
		15q21.1	1.68
		15q21.2	1.59
		15q21.3	1.47
		15q22	1.07
		15q23	0.98
		15q24	0.77
		15q25.1	0.64
		15q25.2	0.58
		15q25.3	0.46
		15q26.1	0.28
		15q26.2	0.12
		15q26.3	0.00
16p11.1	1.10	16q11	1.61
16p11.2	0.91	16q12.1	1.47
16p12.1	0.84	16q12.2	1.32
16p12.2	0.75	16q13	1.16
16p12.3	0.65	16q21	0.97
16p13.11	0.57	16q22.1	0.77
16p13.12	0.48	16q22.2	0.72
16p13.13	0.34	16q22.3	0.58
16p13.2	0.23	16q23.1	0.42
16p13.3	0.00	16q23.2	0.34
		16q23.3	0.29
		16q24	0.00
17p11.1	0.94	17q11.1	2.25
17p11.2	0.61	17q11.2	2.10
17p12	0.45	17q12	2.00
17p13.1	0.31	17q21.1	1.83
17p13.2	0.24	17q21.2	1.75
17p13.3	0.00	17q21.31	1.55
		17q21.32	1.45
		17q21.33	1.33
		17q22	1.18
		17q23.1	1.05
		17q23.2	—
		17q24.1	0.93
		17q24.2	0.75
		17q24.3	0.58
		17q25.1	0.35
		17q25.2	0.28
		17q25.3	0.00
18p11.1	0.67	18q11.1	1.86
18p11.2	0.22	18q11.2	1.58
18p11.31	0.10	18q12.1	1.37
18p11.32	0.00	18q12.2	1.25
		18q12.3	1.12
		18q21.1	0.86
		18q21.2	0.72

Chromosome Band (Short Arm)	Distance of Interband Border to Telomere	Chromosome Band (Long Arm)	Distance of Interband Border to Telomere
		18q21.31	0.61
		18q21.32	0.57
		18q21.33	0.55
		18q22.1	0.40
		18q22.2	0.32
		18q22.3	0.25
		18q23	0.00
19p11	1.11	19q11	1.36
19p12	0.87	19q12	1.14
19p13.11	0.66	19q13.11	0.99
19p13.12	0.54	19q13.12	0.93
19p13.13	0.46	19q13.13	0.76
19p13.2	0.34	19q13.2	0.69
19p13.3	0.00	19q13.31	0.61
		19q13.32	0.56
		19q13.33	0.50
		19q13.41	0.26
		19q13.42	—
		19q13.43	0.00
20p11.1	0.87	20q11.1	1.30
20p11.21	0.75	20q11.21	1.18
20p11.22	0.68	20q11.22	1.07
20p11.23	0.55	20q11.23	0.96
20p12.1	0.41	20q12	0.84
20p12.2	0.36	20q13.11	0.76
20p12.3	0.23	20q13.12	0.65
20p13	0.00	20q13.13	0.42
		20q13.2	0.28
		20q13.31	0.25
		20q13.32	0.18
		20q13.33	0.00
21p11		21q11.1	1.16
21p12		21q11.2	1.12
21p13		21q21.1	0.74
		21q21.2	0.67
		21q21.3	0.57
		21q22.11	0.44
		21q22.12	0.38
		21q22.13	0.32
		21q22.2	0.24
		21q22.3	0.00
22p11		22q11.1	1.24
22p12		22q11.21	1.06
22p13		22q11.22	0.97
		22q11.23	0.90
		22q12.1	0.81
		22q12.2	0.69
		22q12.3	0.59
		22q13.1	0.43
		22q13.2	0.34
		22q13.31	0.24
		22q13.32	0.18
		22q13.33	0.00

Source: Adapted with permission from Daniel, A (1985). The size of prometaphase chromosome segments. *Clinical Genetics*, **28**, 216–224 © Blackwell Publishing Ltd., Oxford.

Index

CPSIA information can be obtained
at www.ICGtesting.com
Printed in the USA
LVOW04s0223180516

488770LV00006B/20/P

9 780195 305272